THE
EVERYTHING®
GUIDE TO PREGNANCY
NUTRITION & HEALTH

Dear Reader,

Congratulations! Whether you are planning to become pregnant, or have already seen the life-changing positive pregnancy test result, your search for information to help you live the healthiest life during this especially important time is something you should take pride in! Before, during, and after your pregnancy, the choices you make about what you do and how you live have profound impacts on you and your baby. Knowing as much as you can about the "good," the "bad," the "right," and the "wrong" while pregnant can help you make the right decisions, and find peace in knowing that you are doing the best you can for your baby and yourself.

As a mom of three, I know firsthand that every pregnancy is different. As a personal trainer and fitness nutrition specialist who specializes in pre- and postnatal health, I know that every pregnancy is different. Luckily, though, there are healthy habits every woman can implement while pregnant that can promote a healthy pregnancy, a healthy mom, and a healthy baby. My goal is to offer answers, advice, and direction in a time that can be one of excitement, but also concern. In this book, I am happy to share information that has helped women like myself make decisions about fitness, nutrition, and life that have made for a healthier, happier experience before, during, and after their wonderful bundle of joy arrives!

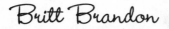

Britt Brandon

Welcome to the EVERYTHING® Series!

These handy, accessible books give you all you need to tackle a difficult project, gain a new hobby, comprehend a fascinating topic, prepare for an exam, or even brush up on something you learned back in school but have since forgotten.

You can choose to read an Everything® book from cover to cover or just pick out the information you want from our four useful boxes: e-questions, e-facts, e-alerts, and e-ssentials.

We give you everything you need to know on the subject, but throw in a lot of fun stuff along the way, too.

We now have more than 400 Everything® books in print, spanning such wide-ranging categories as weddings, pregnancy, cooking, music instruction, foreign language, crafts, pets, New Age, and so much more. When you're done reading them all, you can finally say you know Everything®!

QUESTION

Answers to
common questions

FACT

Important snippets
of information

ALERT

Urgent
warnings

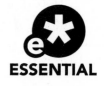

ESSENTIAL

Quick
handy tips

PUBLISHER Karen Cooper

MANAGING EDITOR, EVERYTHING® SERIES Lisa Laing

COPY CHIEF Casey Ebert

ASSOCIATE PRODUCTION EDITOR Mary Beth Dolan

ACQUISITIONS EDITOR Lisa Laing

DEVELOPMENT EDITOR Brett Palana-Shanahan

EVERYTHING® SERIES COVER DESIGNER Erin Alexander

THE
EVERYTHING®
GUIDE TO
PREGNANCY
NUTRITION &
HEALTH

From preconception to post-delivery, all you need to know about pregnancy nutrition, fitness, and diet!

Britt Brandon, CFNS, CPT with Dr. Heather Rupe

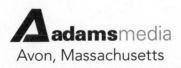
adamsmedia
Avon, Massachusetts

For my wonderful children, Lilly, Lonni, and JD.
And for every mom and mom-to-be who shares the amazingly unique and
precious love for their children that can be compared to no other!

An Everything® Series Book.
Everything® and everything.com® are registered trademarks of F+W Media, Inc.

Published by
Adams Media, a division of F+W Media, Inc.
57 Littlefield Street, Avon, MA 02322. U.S.A.
www.adamsmedia.com

ISBN 10: 1-4405-6011-0
ISBN 13: 978-1-4405-6011-8
eISBN 10: 1-4405-6012-9
eISBN 13: 978-1-4405-6012-5

Printed in the United States of America.

10   9   8   7   6   5   4   3   2   1

The information in this book should not be used for diagnosing or treating any health problem. Not all diet and exercise plans suit everyone. You should always consult a trained medical professional before starting a diet, taking any form of medication, or embarking on any fitness or weight-training program. The author and publisher disclaim any liability arising directly or indirectly from the use of this book.

Many of the designations used by manufacturers and sellers to distinguish their product are claimed as trademarks. Where those designations appear in this book and F+W Media was aware of a trademark claim, the designations have been printed with initial capital letters.

This book is available at quantity discounts for bulk purchases.
For information, please call 1-800-289-0963.

Contents

Acknowledgments

First and foremost, my eternal thanks will forever be for Katie Douglas, my amazing Certified Nurse Midwife (CNM) who delivered all three of my beautiful children. While pregnant with my first daughter, I was blessed to have her teach me to embrace everything I would experience in my pregnancy, trust in myself and my body, live my life for my baby, and have faith that my little angel would be a happy, healthy, astounding human being. Through the amazing moments, and the scary ones, she was the rock that my family and I leaned upon for strength and support . . . and we will forever be grateful for this astounding woman who helped us bring our children into this world, and better our lives beyond our wildest dreams!

I could never forget to thank the best pediatrician any mom could ever ask for, Dr. Douglas Bowling. From breastfeeding to first foods, healthy activity ideas and beyond, we have been so very lucky to have such a wonderful doctor help us understand the best ways to keep our children happy and healthy. We count our blessings each and every day to have had a pediatrician who seems to have the perfect answer all the time, gives us the best ideas to help our children thrive, and has taught us to always trust our instincts . . . since day one!

To Jimmy, Lilly, Lonni, and JD, who have made becoming a mom the best experience of my life! I learn something about you (and myself!) every day, and couldn't imagine a better life than the one I have with you guys! I love you!

The Top 10 Things You Need to Know to Have the Healthiest Pregnancy Possible

1. The foods you choose to consume while pregnant can either provide or deprive your body and your baby of important nutrients that are essential for health.

2. The exercise you engage in daily helps develop all of your baby's systems, as well as the proper functioning of the brain.

3. Many of the common discomforts that are experienced during pregnancy can be alleviated through diet, exercise, and lifestyle habits.

4. Certain exercises should not be performed through all trimesters. Knowing which exercises are recommended and not for each trimester can help you maintain a perfect workout routine that maximizes benefits and minimizes risk.

5. You can keep your immune system strong enough to fight off illnesses throughout pregnancy by making simple healthy choices about your diet, physical activity regimen, and day-to-day habits.

6. Some of the most severe cases of morning sickness can be alleviated with nutritious choices. By knowing how, when, and what you should be eating to minimize digestive discomforts, you can minimize or avoid the queasiness and uneasiness of morning sickness.

7. Allow for maximum blood flow throughout your body and to your baby by sleeping on your left side while pregnant.

8. Engaging in regular physical activity while pregnant can prepare your body for a shorter, less intense, more successful labor and delivery.

9. Stress and anxiety while pregnant can create a terrible environment for both mom and baby. By making certain simple changes to your everyday life, you can easily improve your mood and find a balance!

10. "Bouncing back" physically, mentally, and emotionally after birth is a lot easier if you have an idea of what to expect and start planning and preparing long before baby even arrives.

Introduction

YEARS AGO, PREGNANCY WAS considered a time when women were expected to let themselves go: indulge in foods they craved and limit or refrain from exercise altogether. Weight gain was thought to be a sad and inevitable consequence of the pregnant "condition," and the body of a mother was nothing to which the vain would aspire. While healthy eating and fitness habits were pushed to the wayside, unhealthy habits like smoking, drinking, and a sedentary lifestyle remained the same while pregnant, and that was just the way it was.

Things have changed since those times . . . drastically! Today, in the modern age of technology, research, and longitudinal studies, we have the privilege of having information about pregnancy that was never available to prior generations, thus the view of pregnancy has transformed the dismissive perception of generations past to one in which women are able to do all they can to remain healthy and promote the healthy growth of their unborn baby. The pregnant "condition" is no longer considered a period of time when women are too fragile to engage in activity, too hungry to watch what they eat, or completely oblivious to lifestyle habits during pregnancy that affect both mom and baby while pregnant and well beyond. Today's pregnant women are wanting for the knowledge they can put to use in hopes of delivering the healthiest baby possible . . . and improving their own health to watch that baby grow for as long as possible! From participating in prenatal exercise programs to consuming the healthiest foods that boast loads of vitamins growing babies need, pregnant women are taking control of their pregnancies and being the best moms from conception simply by living their healthiest lives while pregnant . . . and it's not difficult.

Luckily, modern medicine and amazing advancements in technology have allowed pregnancies to be more "carefree" in that you can (literally!) see and hear almost everything about your baby nearly from conception, helping to put minds at ease when it comes to possible complications, questions, or concerns. From the peace of mind that comes from knowing all is well with mom and baby, pregnant women are now able to focus on the nutrition, physical activity, and day-to-day decisions that have been proven time and again to improve the quality of the pregnancy experience (for mom and baby!). While there are always limitations that women should remain aware of while pregnant, exercise is widely accepted and promoted for pregnant women . . . even up until the day of delivery! Clean, minimally processed foods that provide immense nutrition are not only being prioritized in pregnant diets because of their nutritional value but also because of the countless ways those clean foods can act as natural healers and health boosters for both mom and baby.

Embracing the lifestyle that promotes healthy choices is not a difficult one for expectant moms. Knowing that your choices will have a direct impact on the health and quality of life you bestow upon your child is more than enough to make most moms opt for the healthier alternative anytime. For even the most novice of health nuts, newest to exercise, or "go-against-the-grain" lifestyle liver, the small changes you can make to improve your health while pregnant can make a transition to your healthiest life far easier than you'd expect . . . with benefits that will pay off for a lifetime, literally!

CHAPTER 1

Why Pre-Pregnancy Health Matters

One of the easiest ways to ensure you have the healthiest pregnancy possible is to make sure you live healthfully before you even conceive. From maximizing your fertility to implementing healthy lifestyle changes, and choosing your health-care provider to addressing current health problems, the measures you take *before* becoming pregnant can have as profound an impact on your health and the health of your baby as those you take *while* you're pregnant. Luckily, there are a few things you can do to drastically improve your pre-pregnancy health, and each will increase your chances of having a healthy pregnancy, a healthy baby, and a healthier, happier you!

Getting the Green Light

Before you become pregnant, you should know that many questions will arise throughout your pregnancy that you'll be running past your doctor for approval or advice. Since you'll be getting his or her stamp of approval on most things you do for the next year, be sure you find a doctor who makes you feel comfortable if you have questions, want information, or have certain preferences during your pregnancy. When you meet with a medical professional prior to becoming pregnant, you can be sure you are taking the necessary care to ensure you have a healthy pregnancy from conception through delivery. You'll have a chance to ask questions about fertility, conception, and pregnancy. And your physician can help you determine whether you're physically ready for conceiving and pregnancy.

Ideally, your prenatal care should begin before you even become pregnant. According to the U.S. Centers for Disease Control and Prevention, almost 4 million American women give birth each year. Nearly one-third of them will experience some type of pregnancy-related complication. Women who do not seek adequate prenatal care increase their risk for complications that may go undetected or are not dealt with soon enough. This can lead to serious consequences for the mother and/or baby. It's never too early to start prenatal care.

FACT

If you follow a strict vegetarian or vegan diet or participate in strenuous exercise such as long-distance running, your levels of key nutrients and hormones may be affected. Prescription medications, weight-loss diets, anemia, and other health issues also affect these levels, so you should talk to your doctor before trying to get pregnant.

Your doctor can do a thorough physical exam and can explain how pregnancy might affect you as an individual. Your doctor can address any current health issues you may have and discuss with you how it may affect your pregnancy. She can review any medications you are taking and make any changes necessary. She can also make sure you are up to date on immunizations, test you for HIV and other sexually transmitted diseases, and measure your immunity to certain childhood diseases such as chicken pox and rubella. It is a smart idea to have these tests done before you get pregnant to make sure you are in good health. Your prenatal checkup is also a chance to ask any questions you may have.

Choosing a Health-Care Provider

Choosing your health-care provider—and the hospital where you'll have your baby—can be one of the most important decisions you make for you and your baby. Women who are planning to become pregnant are typically cared for by either a board-certified obstetrician/gynecologist (OB/GYN), a family practitioner, or a certified nurse-midwife (CNM). Your health-care provider might be your current OB/GYN or family doctor (if he specializes in obstetrics), or you may want to take this chance to switch doctors if you are not completely comfortable with your present one. Choose a health-care professional who is caring enough to spend a few extra minutes with you to talk about preconception care. If you know which hospital you'll be using, talk to a labor and delivery nurse who works there. No one knows OB/GYNs better than the nurses they work with. The recommendation of family members, friends, and insurance companies can be helpful as well.

Demystifying the Titles

Obstetricians (OB) are doctors who specialize in pregnancy and childbirth. These doctors may or may not also be gynecologists (GYN), who are doctors specializing in women's health care. If your doctor is board certified, you will see the letters FACOG (Fellow of the American Congress of Obstetrics and Gynecology) following her name.

A certified nurse-midwife (CNM) is an advanced-practice nurse who specializes in women's health care, including prenatal care, labor and delivery, and postpartum care for "normal" pregnancies. Most midwives in the United States are CNMs. They have at least a bachelor's degree, and some may have a master's or doctoral degree. Certification means the nurse-midwife has completed both nursing and midwifery training and has passed national and state licensing exams to become certified. Midwives are now licensed to practice in all states, and many work in conjunction with doctors. About 96 percent of CNM-assisted births occur in hospitals. Certified midwives are not registered nurses, but otherwise they meet the same qualifications as a CNM. Currently, only the State of New York recognizes this certification as sufficient for licensure. If you choose a midwife to perform the delivery, make sure to ask about that midwife's credentialing process. Also find out who is supervising her in your care and the delivery of your baby.

ESSENTIAL

CNM-attended births are becoming much more popular. In fact, the American College of Nurse-Midwives estimates that from 1989 to 2000, the number of CNM-attended births increased by almost 125 percent, and by 2010, nearly 20 percent of deliveries were nurse-midwife assisted.

It is up to you to make an educated and informed decision about who will care for you and your baby during pregnancy, so do your research. If you are considered higher risk due to your personal health and/or personal or family health history or there is reason to anticipate complications during your pregnancy or childbirth, you may need to choose a doctor who specializes in your condition. Your OB/GYN should be able to help you pinpoint risk factors and refer you to a specialist if necessary. No matter whom you choose, it is important to make your decision and make a prenatal appointment as soon as possible.

Maximizing Fertility

Do you want to improve your chances for becoming pregnant? With the exception of fertility issues that would require medical intervention, you can take control of maximizing your fertility with a few lifestyle changes that, when implemented early on, will improve your chances of conceiving. Your health and well-being, quality of diet, and healthy or unhealthy habits all increase or decrease your chances of becoming pregnant. If you take the time to focus on improving your overall health, your reproductive health will benefit, too.

Fertility and Nutrition

For both women and men, there is a definite link between nutrition and fertility. Eating a well-balanced, nutritious diet boosts your chances of getting pregnant and having a healthy baby. You should begin making changes to your eating habits at least three months to a year before planning to get pregnant to ensure your body has all of the nutrients it needs to create and sustain a healthy baby.

ALERT

Keep in mind that some herbs on the market can actually decrease fertility. St. John's wort, for instance, can decrease sperm motility in men. Do your research and speak with your doctor before taking any herbal supplement.

Certain vitamins and minerals, such as vitamins C and E, zinc, and folic acid, are crucial for creating healthy sperm. Several studies have indicated that deficiencies in zinc can impede both female and male fertility. You should maintain the dietary reference intake (DRI) of 8 mg per day for women over eighteen years and 11 mg per day for men over eighteen to help keep your reproductive system functioning properly. Men who are deficient in folate have been shown to experience a lower number and poorer quality of sperm. Being deficient in certain nutrients may also affect a woman's menstrual periods, which makes it more difficult to predict when she is ovulating and the best time for her to conceive. Maintaining a diet that includes all of the food groups and living a healthier lifestyle will ensure the most favorable reproductive functioning.

Fertility-Promoting Herbs

Herbs have been used for many years to treat all types of health conditions, and today they are increasingly popular as fertility enhancers. Some of the most popular herbs used for promoting fertility include vitex agnus, black cohosh, dong quai, licorice, Korean ginseng, and pycnogenol. If you are interested in trying natural fertility-enhancing herbs, you should always seek the advice of your health-care provider before taking any new supplement, regardless of whether it is "natural" or not. Many health-care professionals are hesitant about herbs, which are not currently regulated by the FDA (Food and Drug Administration) or the scrutiny of clinical studies. In addition, many factors can affect their potency.

Fertility-Inhibiting Habits

Evidence shows that quitting bad habits such as alcohol, smoking, drug use, and caffeine can increase your chances of conceiving. You should begin to make these healthier lifestyle changes at least three months to a year before you plan to conceive to ensure your body is free of harmful substances.

Keep in mind that, when it comes to fertility, a healthy lifestyle is just as important for men as for women. Sperm can be affected by alcohol, tobacco, drug use, and caffeine as much as a woman's eggs. Some research suggests that certain bad habits can contribute to lower sperm counts and slower sperm motility. So, if conception is a common goal, both the future-mom and the future-dad should focus on changing lifestyle habits for the better in preparation for conception, pregnancy, and parenthood.

Optimizing Prenatal Health

Before becoming pregnant, it is imperative to evaluate some aspects of your lifestyle and decide whether or not they are conducive to a healthy pregnancy. If you engage in certain behaviors that will be harmful during pregnancy, do your best to eliminate them prior to conception. Even while trying to conceive, you should take care with what you do and how you live; chances are you won't find out you're pregnant until a few weeks after you've conceived, and those first weeks are crucial to a baby's development.

FACT

Most of a baby's major organs form very early in pregnancy. Birth defects and other problems can occur before a woman has missed her first period or knows she is pregnant. You can lower the risk of birth defects and problems with pregnancy by making healthy nutritional choices before you even get pregnant.

Nutrition

There are several dietary guidelines that everyone should follow, but there are also specific guidelines for women who are planning to become pregnant. In the months before a woman becomes pregnant, her nutritional intake can be a key factor in the outcome of the pregnancy. The foods she eats and the vitamins and minerals she takes will help ensure that both she and her baby have the nutrients required right from the very start of the pregnancy.

The key to a healthy pregnancy diet is to plan ahead. First, work to improve your diet. You, as well as your partner, need to follow a well-balanced, healthy diet. Meals should be spaced evenly throughout the day and should provide foods from all of the food groups. If you are not sure how to go about eating healthier, now is the perfect time to explore all possible options.

Alcohol

Drinking alcohol during pregnancy can cause both mental and physical birth defects in babies and may result in deformities, social or learning problems, and sometimes death. There is no safe level of alcohol during pregnancy, and it should be completely avoided. That includes the time you are trying to conceive, since you may be pregnant before you realize it. According to recent studies, women who drink alcohol while trying to conceive, even in small amounts, may reduce their chances of becoming pregnant.

Alcohol-related birth defects are more likely to result from the intake of alcohol during the first trimester, when the brain and many of the baby's organs are developing. Growth problems are likely to result from drinking alcohol in the third trimester. Drinking at any stage of the pregnancy can affect the brain. Drinking alcohol can also increase the risk of miscarriage, low birth weight, and stillbirth babies as well as fetal alcohol syndrome. If you are having a problem with drinking, you should seek professional help.

Tobacco

Cigarette smoking or any other kind of tobacco use can be very hazardous throughout your pregnancy. Smoking has been proven to cause miscarriages and preterm delivery, as well as infant death. Smoking can cause low birth weight, asthma in infants and young children, SIDS (sudden infant death syndrome), and other respiratory diseases. People who smoke inhale nicotine and carbon monoxide, both of which can travel through the placenta directly to the baby. This can prevent the fetus from receiving the oxygen and the nutrients it needs to grow and develop properly. Secondhand smoke can be just as hazardous and should be avoided when possible. After pregnancy, it is important to remember that your breast milk often contains what is in your body. If you smoke while breastfeeding, your baby can ingest the nicotine in your milk.

FACT

According to the American Lung Association, "Smoking during pregnancy accounts for an estimated 20 to 30 percent of low birth-weight babies, up to 14 percent of preterm deliveries, and some 10 percent of all infant deaths."

It will not protect your baby if you merely cut down on your smoking or switch to lower-tar cigarettes. Women must quit smoking while trying to conceive, while pregnant, and while breastfeeding. This can be the perfect time to stop smoking for life and help decrease your risk of developing future tobacco-related health problems, such as cancer and heart disease. Quitting smoking can take time, so get started well before you begin trying to conceive to ensure the healthiest start for baby and a healthier life for you.

Caffeine

The risk of caffeine intake during pregnancy is a controversial issue. Still, most experts agree that you should cut back on your caffeine consumption while trying to conceive and while you are pregnant. That doesn't mean you have to completely cut out caffeine, but you should cut down. Most research shows that it is safe to drink coffee or other caffeinated beverages during pregnancy as long as you consume less than three cups, or about 300 mg of caffeine per day (per the American Dietetic Association).

Consumption of more than 300 mg per day has been associated with a possible decrease in fertility and an increased risk of miscarriage or low birth-weight babies. If you are a caffeine junkie, cutting back or cutting out caffeine can be difficult and may cause headaches and fatigue. If you cut back gradually, and work to have it under control by the time you are ready to conceive, you may find it easier to calm or quit your caffeine habit more successfully.

Drug Use

It is crucial that while trying to conceive, women and their partners avoid recreational drugs such as marijuana, cocaine, and other illegal drugs, and it is especially important for the mother to avoid them during pregnancy and breastfeeding. Many recreational drugs are highly addictive, and users may need professional help to kick the habit for good. Most of these drugs can reach the fetus by crossing the placenta and can also be passed through breast milk.

Studies show that using marijuana during pregnancy can result in low birth weight, malformations, poor growth, and fetal neurological problems. The male sperm can also be affected by using this drug. It can take one month for the drug to be completely out of the body, so both partners should quit using any drugs at least a month before even trying to conceive.

The message is simple: If you want to have a healthy baby and a healthy pregnancy, illicit recreational drugs have no place in your life. These drugs have no place in the environment of an infant, and the time to kick these habits is before you even attempt to conceive. Be honest with your doctor—if you are a drug user (habitual or recreational), let him know so that you can get the help that you need.

Your Pre-Pregnancy Weight

Being either overweight or underweight before and during pregnancy can cause problems. Before pregnancy, being significantly over- or underweight has been shown to interfere with ovulation and fertility. Your goal should be to reach a healthy weight or be as close as possible before you conceive.

Being overweight can increase your risk for high blood pressure and gestational diabetes as well as increase the risk of some birth defects. Researchers from the U.S. Centers for Disease Control and Prevention have found a link between pre-pregnancy obesity and the increased risk of neural tube birth defects, including spina bifida. Being overweight but not obese at the time of conception resulted in increased risks of having a child with heart defects or more than one unrelated birth defect.

Underweight women increase the risk of having a low birth-weight baby and a premature delivery. If a woman is underweight due to under-eating, she may not be supplying her body with all the nutrients she needs for a healthy pregnancy, a healthy baby, or healthy motherhood to follow.

Existing Health Problems

If you are currently being treated for a chronic health problem such as diabetes, high blood pressure, thyroid disease, systemic lupus, seizure disorder, inflammatory bowel disease, asthma, heart problems, migraines, or any other condition, you should speak with your doctor before you try to conceive to understand how your health could affect your pregnancy. Your doctor may need to refer you to a specialist and/or change or eliminate certain medications to reduce any possible risk to the fetus. You may have to be much more vigilant about managing your condition and make sure your condition is well under control before you become pregnant.

In addition, you should ensure that all regular medical screening is up to date before you try to conceive. This may include annual pap smears, mammograms (for women over thirty-five), cholesterol screening, and diabetic screening. This should include your partner also. Making sure you are both healthy before you try to conceive can increase your chances of becoming pregnant.

Family History

Some conditions or diseases are genetic, recurring throughout some family histories. Examples include hemophilia (a blood disorder), sickle-cell anemia, cystic fibrosis, Tay-Sachs, thalassemia (or Cooley's anemia), celiac disease, Gaucher disease, Canavan disease, Niemann-Pick disease, and some birth defects. If you or your partner has a family history of a significant genetic disorder, and you suspect that either of you may be a carrier, then genetic testing may be advised. A carrier does not necessarily have the disorder but does carry a gene that could be passed on to the next generation. You should discuss your concerns with your doctor or health-care provider before you get pregnant.

CHAPTER 2

Elements of Great Health

When it comes to preparing your body for pregnancy and motherhood, becoming as healthy as possible as early as possible is absolutely essential! Your health should be your top priority. Decorating the baby's room and planning the baby shower can wait until later, but the time for becoming your healthiest self is now! Starting small and learning as much as you can about becoming your healthiest self can help you achieve optimal prenatal health in no time.

The Impact of Quality Nutrition

The quality of your diet will make or break your health. Your body depends on the food you provide for fueling your body's system functioning, optimizing your immune defenses, providing energy, restoring necessary nutrients to cells in need, and maintaining a body and brain that function in a way to provide you with a happy and healthy life. With pregnancy, your body's responsibilities are multiplied! Your pregnant body has to provide all that you need before becoming pregnant, plus the essentials your baby needs to grow and develop, and everything necessary to provide a successful labor, delivery, and postpartum experience. You can't expect your body to be able to do all of that on a diet of fast food and soda. Eating a diet of natural, whole, "not-messed-around-with" foods that contain rich stores of vitamins and minerals in a wide variety will ensure your body, brain, and baby will have everything necessary to be as healthy as possible during pregnancy and beyond.

The Dietary Guidelines for Americans

The Dietary Guidelines for Americans are made up of ten basic principles for healthy eating. The guidelines are meant to provide sound advice to help people make food choices for a healthy, active life. Following the guidelines will ensure that your eating habits measure up. Therefore, understanding the dietary guidelines should be your first step to making sure you are consuming a diet that is optimal to a healthy pregnancy.

The dietary guidelines follow an easy-to-remember "ABC" organization. Each of the three main topics (Aim for Fitness, Build a Healthy Base, and Choose Sensibly) includes several important points.

The first topic, Aim for Fitness, points out the importance of good physical health:

1. Aim for a healthy weight.
2. Be physically active each day.

The second topic, Build a Healthy Base, gives basic pointers on healthy eating:

3. Let the USDA's MyPlate guidelines influence your food choices.
4. Choose a variety of grains daily, especially whole grains.
5. Choose a variety of fruits and vegetables daily.
6. Keep food safe to eat.

The third topic, Choose Sensibly, provides advice on eating for general health:

7. Choose a diet that is low in saturated fat and cholesterol and moderate in total fat.
8. Choose beverages and foods to moderate your intake of sugars.
9. Choose and prepare foods with less salt.
10. If you drink alcoholic beverages, do so in moderation.

The Dietary Guidelines for Americans are published by the U.S. Department of Agriculture (USDA) and the U.S. Department of Health and Human Services. The guidelines are updated every five years. To be on the cutting edge of good health, look for updated versions as they become available.

Making the Change: Changing Your Eating Habits

Let's say that after a review of the USDA's dietary guidelines, you have determined that your nutritional intake is not up to par. Don't worry—there is time to make some changes. The key is to make only a few changes at a time. Trying to change your entire diet at one time can be frustrating and discouraging. Start with simple goals—such as eating at least three meals a day, eating two servings of fruit per day, drinking eight glasses of water each day, or walking thirty minutes three times per week—and work your way up from there. Once you have mastered one set of habits, move on to the next. Be sure your goals are realistic, specific, and attainable. "Eat more fruit" is a noble goal, but it might help to make one that's more specific, like "Eat two servings of fruit each day."

Find a way to monitor yourself, such as a food journal. There are also many free apps that can be used to track nutrition and calories. Self-monitoring has been shown to help change a behavior in the desired direction. Keep in mind that it takes at least twenty-one days to actually change a habit—so be patient. Use your food journal or food tracking app to record everything you eat and drink throughout the day; this can help you stay committed to your goal of eating a healthier diet. Record each item down as soon as you have eaten it. That way you won't forget to take note of certain foods at the end of the day. And don't forget to keep track of how much water you drink, too.

Focus on the Healthiest Weight for You

A healthy weight is a realistic weight that is best for you—not necessarily the lowest weight you *think* you should be or the "ideal weight" you feel you should be. People come in all shapes and sizes, so it is impossible to use ideal weights or talk about what a "perfect" body should be. A healthy weight is one that puts you at the least risk for health problems related to your weight. Your doctor can help you to determine if you are at a healthy weight.

If you are not at a healthy weight, it is time to think about how you will get there before you begin trying to conceive. Eating to control your weight and eating for good health are really one and the same. A healthy diet and regular exercise can accomplish both goals. To lose weight, you simply need to eat fewer calories, and for weight gain you need to eat more.

FACT

Women who have *more* than fifteen to twenty pounds to lose, have health problems, or are taking medications on a regular basis should see their doctor before beginning a weight-loss program of any kind to ensure your doctor is aware of your plan and you have had an opportunity to discuss all possible weight-loss programs in advance.

If you are overweight, a safe and healthy weight loss is a deficit of 250 to 1,000 calories per day to lose ½ pound to 2 pounds per week. Losing weight any quicker than that means you are losing muscle mass instead of body fat. To lose 1 pound of fat, you need to burn 3,500 more calories than you take in. In other words, losing 1 pound of fat per week means taking in 500 fewer calories per day from your maintenance diet.

Your main goal should be to lose weight safely and sensibly. There are many different types of programs and options available to you. Take your time to find the method that is most appropriate for you. If you need professional help, a registered dietitian can design a safe and effective program for you to follow; a simple Internet search, browse through the phone book, or referral from your primary care physician or GYN can help you locate an RD in your area.

Once you reach your healthy goal weight, the key is to make it permanent and not begin a continuous cycle of yo-yo dieting (or losing and gaining weight). It is important to have the right motivation to maintain weight. Internal motivators such as health, a healthy pregnancy, increased energy, self-esteem, and feeling in control will increase the chances of lifelong success. The probability of long-term maintenance of goals is enhanced in those who exercise regularly, use social support to maintain their eating and exercise habits, interpret lapses positively as solvable problems, and view their eating and exercise regimens as permanent lifestyle habits rather than temporary measures.

Losing Weight Sensibly

The number of calories you consume and the number of calories you burn each day control your body weight. To lose weight, you need to consume fewer calories than you burn. The most successful way to do this is to become more physically active and moderately decrease the number of calories you eat. To safely lose weight most women, on average, need to consume about 1,200 to 1,400 calories daily, depending on factors such as age and activity level. Try to become physically active by walking or doing some other form of aerobic activity thirty minutes a day most days of the week.

Keep in mind that the *type* of calories you eat is also important. Your calories should come from healthy foods, such as fruits, vegetables, whole grains, fat-free or low-fat dairy products, lean meats, fish, poultry, and legumes. Watching your portion sizes carefully within each food group will help keep you within a moderate calorie level. Keep in mind that a gradual weight loss increases your chances of keeping the weight off. Losing weight on your own does not need to be a difficult task. Follow some of these guidelines to lose weight the smart way:

- Eat no more than 30 percent of your total calories from fat (about 40 grams of fat on a 1,200 calorie diet).
- Include at least five servings of fruit and vegetables in your diet each day as well as whole grains. Fiber can help you feel fuller.
- Choose fat-free and lower-fat products over those containing more fat. But don't forget that fat-free does not mean calorie-free!
- Plan your meals and snacks ahead of time—thinking ahead can save you calories.
- If you scarf down your food, slow down! Eating slower can help you eat less.
- Examine your eating habits by keeping a written journal of what, and when, you eat.
- Expect temptation and plan some alternative strategies ahead of time.
- Weigh yourself once a week. Weighing yourself more frequently can be discouraging because weight fluctuates daily with changes in fluid balance.
- Eat breakfast as well as at least four to six small meals per day to help curb binge eating later in the day.

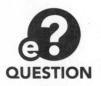

QUESTION

I am overweight and trying to get pregnant. Is it okay to diet?
Strict dieting when planning to become pregnant is not recommended, especially if you leave out certain food groups, eat too few calories, or are on a ketone-promoting diet. Strict dieting can drastically affect the supply of nutrients that is vital for a healthy pregnancy and baby. Women who diet strictly in the years before becoming pregnant may be at higher risk for having low birth-weight babies. If you are concerned about your weight while trying to conceive, stick to a sensible eating plan along with regular exercise. A registered dietitian can help you to design a diet that is right for you.

Gaining Weight Sensibly

If you are under your healthy weight and need to add some pounds, you must do it in a healthy manner. Just because you need to gain weight doesn't mean you should eat whatever you want. You should still eat a healthy diet and just eat more of it. When choosing foods, choose healthy ones with concentrated calories. That way you don't need to increase the portion size as much. These foods can include peanut butter, dried fruits, avocados, nuts, and cheese. Try fortifying soups and casseroles with dry milk powder, or try supplements like Carnation Instant Breakfast to add calories to your intake. Eat more frequently if your appetite is small and avoid drinking fluids close to mealtime so that you don't fill up too easily. A registered dietitian can help with sensible weight gain.

Cardiovascular Exercise

Cardiovascular exercise improves the fitness of your heart and lungs as well as your body's ability to use oxygen. When it comes to selecting a type of cardiovascular exercise that is best for you, keep in mind that all women are different. What works best for one woman may not work for another. Much of the decision will depend on your activity before becoming pregnant. You and your doctor should discuss what would work best for you. It is best to avoid exercises that incorporate excessive bouncing during pregnancy.

ESSENTIAL

Monitor your intensity by monitoring your heart rate while performing cardio exercise. An easy way to monitor your heart rate is to make sure you can always carry on a conversation while you're exercising. If you can't, you are exercising too intensely and should slow down. Modify your pre-pregnancy routine by decreasing both the length and intensity of your workout to avoid fatigue.

Choose activities that are mild to moderate but take longer, as opposed to short-term strenuous exercise. The most comfortable and safe exercises during pregnancy are those that do not require your body to bear extra weight. Good examples include swimming, water aerobics, stationary biking, walking, dancing, yoga, and low-impact aerobics. Jogging and running can be safe during pregnancy, but they are better suited to women who were already doing this type of exercise prior to becoming pregnant.

You could also join a class for expectant moms led by an expert in the prenatal exercise area. These classes can also act as a great support system for you and get you out to meet and socialize with new friends.

Strength Training

Strength training can provide benefits for mom and baby as part of a regular prenatal exercise plan. It can help strengthen and tone muscles as well as build stamina. Women who were not participating in a strength-training program before pregnancy are usually advised to seek advice from a professional fitness specialist who specializes in prenatal fitness to ensure safety before starting a strength-training regimen. Strength training is not appropriate for all pregnant women and should be discussed with your doctor before you begin.

When using weights, it is important to use slow, controlled movements to help avoid injury to loosened joints and ligaments. Machines are generally preferred to free weights during pregnancy because they are more easily controlled. It is advisable to work with lighter weights than you might normally use and to compensate for the lower weight by doing more repetitions. It is important to breathe normally during strength training and avoid holding your breath so your baby continues to receive optimal amounts of oxygen. As with any exercise at this time, discontinue any strength exercise that causes pain or discomfort.

FACT

Avoid exercising the same muscles for two days in a row. Your muscles need time to recover. To see results, you only need to perform strength-training exercises for thirty minutes two to three days per week.

Starting with your second trimester, you should avoid lifting weights while standing. Blood can pool in your legs and cause you to feel lightheaded or dizzy. Avoid lying on a bench to lift weights or being in a position that leaves your abdominal area vulnerable to a falling weight. Use common sense if you plan on weight-training during pregnancy, and discuss your program with your doctor before you begin.

Yoga

Yoga can be a great exercise for flexibility, relaxation, muscle tone, posture, balance, breathing control, and developing concentration. All of these factors can help during pregnancy and again during delivery. Yoga combined with a low-impact cardiovascular exercise such as walking can round out a great exercise program. You can join a pregnancy yoga class or pick up a DVD specifically made for pregnant women.

If you have never tried yoga before, be sure to start at the beginners' level. Yoga can be done at all different intensity levels, but while you are pregnant, you should concentrate on poses that are soothing, gentle, and fun. You want to make sure you avoid positions that require you to lie on your back after the third month. After your belly begins to grow, avoid positions that have you lying face down. As with any exercise program, consult with your doctor before you begin.

ESSENTIAL

One of the essentials of yoga is breathing. In yoga you learn to breathe fully by taking in air slowly through the nose, filling your lungs entirely, and exhaling completely. Learning how to master this type of breathing can be beneficial for pregnancy and in helping you to prepare for labor and delivery.

Some yoga moves can be tricky, so if you feel pain or discomfort, make needed adjustments. Don't hold poses for too long, and move into and out of yoga positions slowly and carefully to avoid any injury or lightheadedness. As you become larger in your third trimester, use a chair or other sturdy prop for support to avoid losing your balance. Equipment such as blocks and straps can help you to more easily move through different poses with better stability. Avoid poses that are difficult and that you may not be familiar with as well as those that stretch the abdominal muscles too much. It is important to be extra careful because you are more prone to tearing and/or straining muscles and ligaments while pregnant.

Kegel Exercises

Kegel exercises can be very helpful once you get to the delivery room. Kegels, or pelvic-floor muscle exercises, are internal exercises that can be done to help strengthen the muscles that control your urethra, bladder, uterus, and rectum. This exercise strengthens the pelvic floor so that during delivery you are able to push more efficiently. Strengthening these muscles can also assist your body in recovering more quickly after delivery. They can help with bladder control problems that many women experience after childbirth.

Kegels are done most simply by contracting and holding the muscles that are used to stop the flow of urine. Try to do Kegels in sets of ten, and work up to three to four sets about three times each day. Start out slow, and work your way up as these muscles become stronger. Make sure you are doing the exercises correctly. If you are not sure, ask your doctor.

Keep Your Immunity Strong

Do what you can to take care of yourself and avoid infections. Some infections can be harmful to the fetus, so keep up your resistance. You can do this by washing your hands, keeping your distance from people around you who are sick, and staying away from unsafe foods. Ensuring that you eat the healthiest foods possible will also help you maintain a strong immune system by delivering the essential vitamins and minerals your body needs in order to function at its best.

When you feel that you're pushing yourself too much and you notice that you're feeling overwhelmed, stressed, undernourished, or overly tired, your immunity can be in danger. Stress, lack of sleep, a deficiency in certain nutrients, and a schedule that doesn't allow for "down time" can come together to create a perfect storm that can weaken your immune system and make you susceptible to illnesses and disease that your body would otherwise be able to fend off when healthy.

Even if you have the best intentions and take optimal care of yourself, you may not be able to completely protect yourself from catching a cold or the flu virus while you are pregnant. Though you may decrease your chances, you are still vulnerable. Because of changes in your immune system during pregnancy, symptoms from colds and/or the flu can persist longer than normal. Pregnancy also increases the risk of complications from the flu and other viruses. Call your doctor immediately if you come down with any type of illness. Some viruses, such as those that cause chicken pox or fifth disease, can be more dangerous if contracted during pregnancy. If you come in contact with anyone who is infected with these or any other contagious illness, contact your doctor immediately.

Protecting Yourself

Eating a healthy diet (one that includes all the food groups in proper amounts), drinking plenty of water, and exercising regularly can definitely decrease your chances of becoming sick while you are pregnant. However, you may need to take additional steps and be extra careful during the cold and flu season. Be careful of the contact you have with family or friends, including children, who may be sick. Wash your hands regularly to lessen the risk of coming in contact with virus germs, especially in public places. Make your visits to crowded places less frequent, as they can be a breeding ground for germs.

If you will be more than three months pregnant during the flu season, you should talk to your doctor about getting a flu shot. If you have medical problems such as diabetes that can increase your risk of complications from the flu, talk to your doctor about getting a flu shot, no matter what trimester you are in.

ALERT

Because flu shots are actually made from inactivated viruses, many doctors consider the flu shot safe during all stages of pregnancy. There is no harm to the baby if the vaccine is given while you are breastfeeding. Speak to your doctor before getting a flu shot.

Emotional Health

Although physical wellness and mental health are often perceived as two separate things, the truth is that the mind and body are inextricably linked and what impacts one usually affects the other as well. This connection is particularly strong in pregnancy as the rapid physical changes taking place alter the biochemical balance of the body and brain. Pregnancy is also a precursor to one of the biggest life-changing events there is—the arrival of a baby—and that alone is enough to stir up new and unexpected feelings.

The hormonal changes that occur in pregnancy can have you feeling weepy one minute and irritable the next. The emotions you experience, especially the negative ones, can be detrimental to your growing child. Depression, stress, and anxiety may alter your eating and sleeping patterns, robbing you and baby of the nutrients and rest you need. Clinical studies have found that depression and stress also have a direct impact on fetal growth and infant development.

ALERT

If you're feeling hopeless, sad, or tired; having trouble sleeping; or losing interest in things that once gave you pleasure, you may be experiencing antepartum depression. Research has linked depression during pregnancy to preterm delivery, lower birth weight, developmental problems in infancy, and a 50 percent chance of developing postpartum depression. Don't wait; talk to your provider about treatment options today.

If you are feeling blue, you aren't alone; one in ten women experiences depressive symptoms at some point in her pregnancy. Frequently, women feel guilty if they are feeling depressed or overwhelmed during a period of their lives that is supposed to be joyful, and for that reason many do not seek professional help. If you feel consistent emotional strain of any type, do what's best for you and your baby and speak to someone who can help.

Sleep

Many moms joke that pregnant women should "sleep while they can," suggesting they should get enough sleep while pregnant because sleep may be limited after the baby's birth. Not only is it important to allow yourself the ample time needed to rest, relax, and recover from each day, it is absolutely essential to your physical, mental, and emotional well-being that you fulfill your body's need for sleep as much as possible.

It's been recommended that the average woman get between seven and eight hours of sleep each night. While pregnant, you should sleep for the amount of time *you* need in order to feel your best. While you're asleep, your body is working overtime to use and store nutrients for you and your baby, replenish cells, revive mental functioning, and restore your feelings of restfulness, without any of which you would be exhausted, short-tempered, foggy-minded, and physically weak. Without these essential sleep-restored elements of physical, mental, and emotional well-being, your overall health can suffer immensely. Unable to exercise, being more prone to make poor food choices, and feeling scattered and moody combine for a situation in which no woman would be able to enjoy her pregnancy to the fullest.

Whether you need seven or ten hours in any given twenty-four-hour period, your body's need for sleep is a crucial area for you to focus on. If you spend the time creating a sleep ritual that involves winding-down time to allow your thought processes to calm, making sure your sleep environment is free of distraction, and that your body and mind are able to be comfortable and peaceful once you're in bed and ready for sleep, you can create a routine that allows you to enjoy sleep whether it's a quick nap in the morning or afternoon, or a deep slumber at night.

CHAPTER 3

Clean Up Your Diet

Focusing on the quality of your diet is a big step toward living the healthiest life for you and your baby. Instead of drastically changing your diet, feeling overwhelmed or deprived, and falling back into an unhealthy diet cycle, you can use some easy-to-apply tips to clean up your diet gradually and painlessly. While you are pregnant and eating for two, you should maintain a diet that optimizes the nutritional content of every bite and sip, and minimizes the unhealthy aspects of foods that won't benefit you or your baby.

The "Eating for Two" Myth

Once you become pregnant, you may hear comments like, "Go ahead and eat, you are eating for two now." It is true that you need nutrients through the foods you choose for both you and the healthy development of your baby. Eating plenty of nutritionally dense foods—as opposed to junk that contains calories but very little nutrition—is the way to supply your baby with all the nutrition he needs. On the other hand, you don't need to eat enough calories for two people. In fact, eating too much can cause unnecessary weight gain. At the same time, eating too little may keep your baby from receiving all of the nutrition he needs. The key is to keep a healthy balance.

Calorie needs increase slightly during pregnancy to help support a woman's maternal body changes and the baby's proper growth and development. It is true that your body requires more calories during pregnancy, but "more" here means only a moderate amount. During the first trimester, most physicians recommend no increase in daily caloric intake for women who are of a healthy weight. After the first trimester, you need about 300 calories per day above your maintenance level. That adds up to about 85,000 calories over the nine months that you are pregnant. Calorie needs will be more if you are carrying more than one baby. Your extra daily calorie needs will jump to 500 calories if you breastfeed following pregnancy. It does not take much to consume an extra 300 calories. The key is to choose nutrient-rich foods that contain plenty of lean protein, complex carbohydrates, fiber, vitamins, and minerals for your extra calories. An extra 300 calories can translate to any of the following:

- A 6-ounce baked potato, with skin, topped with 2 ounces of low-fat cheese, ½ cup of broccoli, and ¼ cup of salsa
- ½ cup tuna salad, half a piece of pita bread, lettuce, tomato, with 1 tablespoon low-fat mayo
- 8 ounces skim milk or 8 ounces low-fat yogurt, a banana, and ¼ cup low-fat granola

Max Out Nutrition

Every macronutrient (carbohydrates, proteins, and fats) and micronutrient (vitamins and minerals) is utilized by the body in different ways. Without even one of these essential elements, one or more of the body's systems can pay a heavy price. Each meal and snack you eat should contain foods that supply ample amounts of complex carbohydrates, clean protein, and healthy fats. Vitamins and minerals are plentiful in natural foods, so eating a variety of natural nutritious options should also be a top priority. By including a variety of foods that contain balanced provisions of macronutrients and micronutrients, you can promote optimal system functioning . . . with the added benefit of delicious meals that have a variety of colors, textures, and flavors.

ALERT

Skipping meals during pregnancy can have serious effects on the proper development of the baby. Skipping meals will force the baby to go too long without proper nourishment, and it can sabotage your efforts to consume enough healthy calories each day.

The vibrant colors of foods signify their high content of great, unique nutrition. From blueberries' blue anthocyanins to broccoli's green chlorophyll and phytochemicals, foods you choose to include in your diet should be appealing to the eyes as well as the palate. By focusing your diet on foods that make your plate (or your glass) as colorful as possible, you can benefit from the variety of nutrients contained within each and every food you enjoy.

Eat Every Three to Four Hours

The body's metabolism is designed to run similarly to a car engine. With fuel, you can run, but without fuel, you can't. Expecting your body to run on little or no food for long periods of time would be like expecting your car to drive long distances at high speeds on nothing but fumes. Expecting your body to be able to create a baby healthfully with little or no fuel would be just as absurd! Fueling up your body every three to four hours with quality nutrition will not only deliver the essential nutrients your body and baby need but also promote a speedy metabolism and provide your body with the energy it needs to function properly. As an added benefit, eating every couple of hours helps satisfy hunger longer and keeps cravings and the temptation to binge on unhealthy foods at bay.

ALERT

People who eat most of their calories at night after hours of deprivation have weight gain and other negative, and sometimes serious, consequences. By overloading the metabolism at night, sugar spikes in the blood, digestive enzymes overload when you are in a reclined position, and excessive calories get stored while you sleep rather than utilized. All these troubles can be avoided by simply redistributing calories evenly throughout the day.

While some people skip breakfast or go long hours without eating under the misconception that fewer meals will result in consuming fewer calories, the reality is that dangerous consequences can result from this short-term starvation. When you choose to forego your morning meal, it's not just your health at stake—your baby's development is as well. Eating five or six balanced and somewhat proportionate meals will help ensure your baby is receiving adequate amounts of the vitamins, minerals, and macronutrients he needs around the clock.

When your body is forced to function on little or no food, it turns to a sort of "hibernation mode" and begins to burn its own sources of fuel for energy. Because muscle mass provides more energy pound-per-pound compared to fat, the body burns the meatier muscle mass for fuel *and* starts to store consumed calories in preparation for upcoming "hibernation" periods. Breaking the day's total calories into five or six equal meals and snacks allows your body's metabolism to increase and the bodily systems to run at peak performance.

Water Intake

Water is an essential part of a healthy lifestyle that is just as important as macronutrients and micronutrients. Water acts as your body's transportation system to carry nutrients to your body cells as well as your baby's. Water helps to regulate body temperature through perspiration and by transporting oxygen through the body, carrying waste products away from the body cells, cushioning joints, and protecting body organs. Proper hydration before, during, and after any form of exercise or vigorous activity is a vital component of a healthy pregnancy.

How Much Is Enough?

Pregnant women need extra fluid to support their increased blood volume and for amniotic fluid. Because the body has no provision to store water, the amount of water you lose each day must be continually replaced to maintain proper hydration. During both pregnancy and breastfeeding, women should aim to drink eight to twelve (8-ounce) glasses of water per day. This may increase if you are perspiring in hot weather, when exercising, or if you have any type of fever, diarrhea, or vomiting.

ESSENTIAL

It is normal to get thirsty once in awhile, but if you are excessively thirsty and find yourself drinking large amounts of water, this could be a sign of a medical condition such as diabetes. If you feel you are drinking because of severe thirst, as opposed to a healthy habit, speak to your doctor.

Inadequate water intake can lead to problems like fatigue, muscle weakness, and headaches, just to name a few. For the fetus, dehydration can affect adequate nutrient transport, induce poor waste removal, create too warm an environment, and decrease cushioning. These can all affect fetal growth and development. Being properly hydrated can help to reduce swelling and bothersome constipation.

Staying properly hydrated can help you to feel more energized, give you an improved sense of well-being, provide greater endurance and stamina during physical activity, and improve your digestion and elimination.

The best and easiest way to get your fluids is simply by drinking water. Other fluids that can contribute to your daily intake include fat-free or low-fat milk, club soda, bottled water, vegetable juice, seltzer, and fruit juice. Be careful of drinking too many beverages, such as juice, that are healthy but also pack in a lot of calories. Stay clear of alcohol and most herbal teas, and limit coffee, tea, soft drinks, diet soft drinks, and other caffeinated beverages. If you feel thirsty, your body is telling you that it is already becoming dehydrated, so drink up.

FACT

Water contributes close to 55 to 65 percent of an adult's body weight, and during pregnancy your body's water needs expand substantially. Water is present in every part of your body: 83 percent of blood, 73 percent of muscle, 25 percent of body fat, and even 22 percent of bones are made up of water.

A Good Habit to Have

Like everything else, drinking water should be part of your healthy lifestyle—you should make it a habit. Make a commitment today to start drinking water on a regular basis. You should be in the habit before you even become pregnant. You should start out with a moderate goal and work your way up. It may help to start a water diary on a calendar to keep track of your current intake and your progress. If you need help increasing your water intake, follow some of these helpful tips:

- At work or at home, take water breaks instead of coffee breaks.
- Keep a bottle of water at your desk, on your counter at home, or in your car when traveling so you have it available to sip throughout the day.
- Get in the habit of drinking a glass of water before and with meals and snacks. Besides helping you to stay hydrated, it can help take the edge off of your appetite.
- Use a straw to drink your water. Believe it or not, using a straw can help you drink faster and make a glass of water seem a little more manageable.
- Drink water instead of snacking while watching television or reading a book.
- Keep a two-quart container of water in the refrigerator, and make it your goal to drink it all by the end of the day. This also gives you a constant supply of good, cold water.

Easy on the Salt

While sodium is a very important mineral during pregnancy, be careful not to overdo it. For many people, consuming sodium in moderation means making some dietary and lifestyle changes. A strong preference for salty foods is easily acquired and usually starts at a young age. It is all in what your taste buds get used to.

To help moderate the amount of sodium in your diet, begin to gradually decrease your salt intake, especially if you are accustomed to salty tastes. Eat plenty of fresh or frozen fruits and vegetables as well as fresh foods as opposed to processed, canned, or prepared foods. If you eat frozen convenience foods often, look for products that have less than 800 mg sodium per serving. Choose lower-sodium foods by paying attention to the nutrition facts panel on all packaged foods. Keep in mind that condiments such as ketchup, soy sauce, teriyaki sauce, mustard, pickles, and olives can be high in sodium, so go easy on these.

Meatless Moms-to-Be

Being pregnant does not mean you have to give up your vegetarian lifestyle. However, just as with any other eating style, if you are following a vegetarian diet during pregnancy, you must ensure that you get well-balanced and varied meals. Although the typical vegetarian diet is very low in saturated fat and cholesterol, not all diets are low in calories, total fat, or sugar. Some can also be lacking in other essential vitamins and minerals unless they are properly planned.

Vegetarianism is a type of eating style that is a matter of personal choice. Some people choose to avoid all animal products, while others may choose to consume some animal foods such as eggs and/or dairy products (lacto-ovo vegetarian). There is also a percentage of vegetarians that are vegans, who avoid all animal products. The majority of vegetarians in the United States fit into the lacto-ovo vegetarian category.

Vegetarians are classified into several different categories, as follows:

- **Vegan:** Absolutely no animal foods, including meat, fish, poultry, eggs, honey, milk, or other dairy products. Also, no foods made with any type of animal product, such as refried beans made with lard or baked goods made with eggs.

- **Lacto vegetarian:** Dairy foods permitted, but no other animal foods including eggs and meats (meat, poultry, fish, and seafood).
- **Lacto-ovo vegetarian:** Dairy foods and eggs permitted, but no other animal foods, including meats (meat, poultry, fish, and seafood).
- **Pescatarian:** Fish and seafood are permitted, but no other animal meat.
- **Semi-vegetarian:** A mostly vegetarian diet (lacto-ovo vegetarian), but meat, poultry, or fish is eaten occasionally.

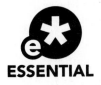

ESSENTIAL

People turn to vegetarian diets for all kinds of reasons, including religious, ethical, environmental, and personal health concerns. For some, vegetarianism is simply a way of eating while for others it is a way of life. There are different types of vegetarian eating styles, and each one differs as to what nutrients may be missing and what adjustments might be necessary to ensure optimal nutritional intake during pregnancy.

Vegetarian Safety During Pregnancy

With careful planning, a vegetarian diet, no matter what the type, can be healthy and safe during pregnancy. By focusing any of the vegetarian diets on consuming high amounts of certain foods like unrefined grains, vegetables, fruits, beans, nuts, and seeds, a pregnant vegetarian can ensure the safest diet, high in a variety of necessary nutrients, needed for mom and baby. Throughout pregnancy, it is absolutely essential to periodically assess your intake of certain nutrients like vitamin B_{12}, calcium, vitamin D, iron, zinc, and protein that are especially important during pregnancy, and make changes as needed.

If you follow a lacto or lacto-ovo vegetarian diet, meaning you include dairy or dairy and eggs in your eating plan, you have fewer nutritional hurdles to get over. If you are vegan, you have to be much more vigilant about consuming all of the essential nutrients you need for a healthy pregnancy. That includes making sure that you consume enough calories recommended for pregnancy. Vegetarians, especially vegans, should keep tabs on their weight gain during pregnancy.

Artificial Sweeteners

Artificial, or nonnutritive, sweeteners are added to all types of foods including gum, candy, sweets, soft drinks, and even some over-the-counter medications. If you are trying to avoid these sweeteners or limit your consumption, read labels closely. Artificial sweeteners that are classified as "generally recognized as safe" are acceptable to use during pregnancy in moderation. However, the use of artificial sweeteners might encourage you to opt out of more nutritious foods. For example, if you drink gallons of diet soft drinks, you may not be drinking other more nutritious beverages such as water, milk, and juice that can be more beneficial. Also, foods with artificial sweeteners are usually lower in calories, and pregnancy is not the time to be eating very low-calorie foods. However, artificial sweeteners can be useful to pregnant women who have diabetes.

Aspartame

Aspartame is an artificial sweetener that is found in popular products such as NutraSweet, Equal, and most diet soft drinks. This sweetener has not been shown to cause birth defects, and the FDA considers moderate use during pregnancy to be safe.

Saccharin

With all of the artificial sweeteners now on the market today, saccharin is much less commonly used. Saccharin is an artificial sweetener that is found in products such as Sweet'N Low and some diet soft drinks as well as some over-the-counter medications. Saccharin was recently removed from the government's list of possible carcinogens after years of research. However, saccharin still carries a warning label until the FDA or congress removes it. Saccharin can cross the placenta and enter the baby's bloodstream. Research has shown that a baby clears saccharin from the bloodstream more slowly than the mother does. Whether this causes harm to the fetus or not is still a controversial issue. Some doctors may ban saccharin from their patient's diets. Because of the controversial and unknown safety of saccharin and unborn babies, it is suggested that saccharin be ingested in moderation if at all during pregnancy.

Acesulfame-K

Acesulfame-K is marketed under the name Sunette. Acesulfame-K has recently been used in the product Pepsi One, which also includes aspartame, as well as candy, baked goods, desserts, and tabletop sweeteners such as Sweet One. The use of acesulfame-K within FDA guidelines appears safe during pregnancy.

Sucralose

Sucralose is one of the newest low-calorie sweeteners on the market and is the generic name for the product called Splenda. It was only approved by the FDA in 1998. This sweetener is actually made from sugar, but unlike sugar, it is not recognized as a carbohydrate during food digestion or absorption. The sweetener is not digested, absorbed, or metabolized for energy, so it does not affect blood sugar or insulin. Instead, sucralose basically passes through the body unchanged. Splenda can be found in many different products and is also packaged as a tabletop sweetener. Sucralose is safe for pregnant women to consume, and as with other sweeteners it is best used in moderation.

Preservatives, Additives, and Chemicals

Many of the foods you eat are full of food additives, such as preservatives, flavor enhancers, food colorings, and even hormones. These additives are used to add color, enhance flavor, sweeten, and preserve food freshness. New additives must pass very rigid government safety tests before they are considered safe for consumers. The U.S. Food and Drug Administration (FDA) is the entity responsible for approving additives used in foods. The FDA sets safety standards, determines whether a substance is safe for its intended use, decides what type of foods the additive can be used in, what amounts it can be used in, and how it must be indicated on food labels.

Some additives are labeled as "Generally recognized as safe" (GRAS) because they have an extensive history of safe use or because existing scientific evidence indicates their safe use in foods. There is an extensive list of GRAS additives, which the FDA and USDA re-evaluate from time to time.

Most food additives are safe during pregnancy unless you have a known reaction or specific allergy to certain food additives. As a pregnant woman, you should get in the habit of reading labels carefully, especially if you are sensitive to any food additives or colorings. If you are concerned about food additives, the best advice is to eat a wide variety of fresh foods. A diet high in whole grains, fresh fruits, fresh vegetables, and fresh meats can help you avoid excessive amounts of some food additives.

MSG

Monosodium glutamate, known as MSG, is used as a flavor enhancer. MSG does not add a flavor of its own to food; instead, it enhances or intensifies the natural salty taste of many processed foods. Although the additive is best known for its use in Chinese food, it is also incorporated into many other processed foods. MSG is made up of sodium and glutamate, or glutamic acid. Glutamic acid is an amino acid that is found naturally in the body and in high protein foods. The FDA classifies MSG as a "generally recognized as safe" additive. Because some people have an adverse reaction to it, the FDA requires all foods that contain MSG to indicate it as an ingredient on the label. In sensitive people, whether pregnant or not, MSG can trigger headaches, nausea, vomiting, sleep disturbances, and dizziness. More severe symptoms include breathing problems, chest pains, and increased blood pressure. Some studies in mice have shown possible birth defects and behavioral problems when MSG is consumed in large amounts, but no correlation has been established for humans. The FDA believes MSG is safe for the majority of the population to consume.

If you are worried about ingesting MSG during pregnancy and how it may affect you and your baby, you should become aware of what foods contain it and limit your intake.

Olestra

Olean, also known as Olestra, is a noncaloric fat substitute that is made of a synthetic mixture of sugar and vegetable oil. Olestra was certified as safe by the FDA in 1996 and was approved for use in snack foods including potato chips, tortilla chips, and crackers. Olestra basically passes through the body undigested. Because it is not absorbed, there is no danger in pregnant women of its reaching the fetus.

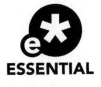

ESSENTIAL

Remember that just because a food contributes no fat, it doesn't necessarily contain zero calories. Foods that contain Olestra will probably not harm you or your baby if eaten in moderation, but there are much better snack choices you can make.

However, there can be some negative effects from eating Olestra. It does interfere with the absorption of the fat-soluble vitamins A, D, E, and K. For that reason, the manufacturer is required to fortify Olestra products with those vitamins. The product also causes mild gastrointestinal discomfort such as diarrhea, gas, abdominal cramping, and greasy stools. The FDA initially required that Olestra products be labeled with a warning of the artificial fat's gastrointestinal effects. Recently, the FDA dropped the requirement because the effects are only mild for most people.

During pregnancy, you probably already deal with plenty of gastrointestinal discomforts. There is no need to compound these problems with foods that contain Olestra. In addition, they provide no real nutritional value. This is a time when you need foods that contain loads of nutrition. There are much better choices when it comes to snacks. Don't get yourself into the habit of snacking on chips, whether they contain fat or not. Instead, get in the habit of snacking on fruits, vegetables, yogurt, and other healthier foods.

CHAPTER 4

Know Your Nutrients

The easiest way to max out the nutrition you consume is to become familiar with the nutrients you have available in your favorite foods. From apples to spinach, smoothies to pasta dishes, you can take your favorite foods and create breakfasts, lunches, dinners, and snacks that are easy and delicious, satisfying, and beneficial, with more essential nutrients than you ever thought possible!

What's in a Serving?

Eating a variety of foods from all of the food groups is the best way to ensure you are getting the calories and nutrients you need. The USDA's MyPlate (*www.choosemyplate.gov*) is a good suggested guideline for pregnant women; it ensures you consume the following minimum number of servings in each food group (about 2,500 calories):

- **Nine servings from the bread, cereal, rice, and pasta group.** Examples of a single serving from this group include a slice of whole-wheat bread, ½ cup cooked cereal, half a bagel, or ½ cup of pasta. Be sure to include whole-grain and whole-wheat starches as well as other starches higher in fiber.
- **Four servings from the vegetable group.** Examples of a single serving from this group include 1 cup of raw leafy vegetables, ½ cup of other vegetables, raw or cooked, or ¾ cup vegetable juice. Choose a variety of vegetables—the darker the color, the more nutrients a vegetable has.
- **Three servings from the fruit group.** Examples of a single serving from this group include a medium apple, a small banana, a small orange, ½ cup chopped fruit, or ¾ cup fruit juice. Choose a variety of fruits daily, as raw fruits are higher in fiber than juices.
- **Three to four servings from the milk, yogurt, and cheese group.** Examples of a single serving from this group include 1 cup of milk or yogurt, 1½ ounces natural cheese, or 2 ounces processed cheese. Use fat-free or low-fat milk, nonfat or low-fat yogurt, and low-fat cheese.
- **Two to three servings (or 6–7 ounces) from the meat, poultry, fish, dry beans, eggs, and nuts group.** Examples of a single serving from this group include 3 ounces poultry, fish, or lean meat; 1 ounce meat = ½ cup cooked dried beans, a whole egg, ½ cup tofu, ⅓ cup nuts, or 2 tablespoons peanut butter. Choose lean meats and trim fat from meat before cooking. With poultry, remove skin. Include cooked dry beans often as the main dish in meals.

Vitamins

Vitamins are known as micronutrients because you need them in much smaller amounts than carbohydrates, proteins, and fats. Even though you need them in smaller amounts, that does not make them any less important. Vitamins are involved in all kinds of functions throughout the body. They don't supply energy directly because they do not provide any calories to the body, but vitamins do regulate many of the processes that produce energy. Although all vitamins are important during pregnancy—and you should concentrate on getting enough of all of them—some deserve special attention. Vitamins fall into two categories: water-soluble and fat-soluble vitamins.

Fat-Soluble Vitamins

The fat-soluble vitamins include vitamins A, D, E, and K. Fat-soluble vitamins dissolve in fat, and they travel throughout the body by attaching to body chemicals made with fat. These vitamins can be stored in the body, so it can be harmful to consume more than you need over a long period of time.

Vitamin A

Vitamin A promotes the growth and the health of cells and tissues for both the mother and the baby. In the form of beta-carotene, vitamin A also acts as a powerful antioxidant. Beta-carotene does not pose any danger to expectant mothers. Your body converts beta-carotene to vitamin A only when the body needs it. The recommended daily allowance (RDA) of vitamin A is measured in micrograms (mcg). In supplements and on nutrition facts panels, it is measured in international units (IU). The need for vitamin A increases only slightly during pregnancy, from 700 to 770 mcg (for women nineteen to fifty years of age).

Vitamin D

Another important fat-soluble vitamin during pregnancy is vitamin D. This vitamin aids in calcium balance and helps your body absorb sufficient calcium for you and your baby. Vitamin D is known as the "sunshine vitamin" because the body can make vitamin D after sunlight hits the skin. It is important to get enough vitamin D throughout your life as a way of helping to avoid osteoporosis (or brittle bone disease). Since vitamin D is stored in the body, too much can be toxic. Excess amounts usually come from supplements and not food or too much sunlight. During pregnancy, women should get 650 IU per day.

Water-Soluble Vitamins

The water-soluble vitamin group consists of the B-complex vitamins and vitamin C. Water-soluble vitamins dissolve in water and are then carried in your bloodstream. Most are not stored in the body in any significant amounts. What your body does not use is excreted through the urine. Since they are not stored in the body, water-soluble vitamins pose less of a risk for toxicity (though moderation is still the best approach). This also means that you need a regular supply from your diet.

Folic Acid

Folic acid is a B vitamin whose main role is to maintain the cell's genetic code or DNA (the cell's master plan for cell reproduction). It also works with vitamin B_{12} to form hemoglobin in red blood cells. Folic acid has gained much attention for its role in reducing the risk for neural tube birth defects, such as spina bifida, in newborn babies. Other risks of folic acid deficiencies include anemia, impaired growth, and abnormal digestive function. It is vital that pregnant women or women of childbearing years consume enough folic acid through food and supplements, especially during the first trimester.

FACT

The B-complex vitamins are a family of vitamins that all work together and have similar functions in health. They include vitamin B_1 (thiamin), vitamin B_2 (riboflavin), niacin, vitamin B_6, folate, vitamin B_{12}, biotin, and pantothenic acid. Most B vitamins help the body to indirectly produce energy within its cells.

Before pregnancy a woman's need for folic acid is 400 mcg per day. During pregnancy, that amount jumps to 600 mcg per day. Recent studies show that to decrease the risk of birth defects, women planning a pregnancy should increase their daily intake of folic acid to 800–1,000 mcg. Most prenatal vitamins contain 800–1,000 mcg to ensure that women fully absorb the amount they need during pregnancy to help decrease the risk of birth defects. Taking too much folic acid through supplements can mask a vitamin B_{12} deficiency and could interfere with some medications. However, some women may need more folic acid with certain medications.

Other B Vitamins

Vitamin B_6 is necessary in helping your body make nonessential amino acids (the building blocks of protein). These nonessential amino acids are used to make necessary body cells. Vitamin B_6 also helps to turn the amino acid tryptophan into niacin and serotonin (a messenger in the brain). In addition to those functions, this vitamin helps produce insulin, hemoglobin, and antibodies that help fight infection. Requirements are increased slightly in pregnancy due to the needs of the baby. The recommended level during pregnancy is 1.9 mg.

Requirements are also increased for vitamin B_{12} during pregnancy to help with the formation of red blood cells. The increase is slight, from 2.4 mcg before pregnancy to 2.6 mcg during pregnancy. This vitamin is found mostly in foods of animal origin, so vegetarians need a reliable source of vitamin B_{12}, such as fortified breakfast cereal or supplements.

Vitamin C

Vitamin C produces collagen, a connective tissue that holds muscles, bones, and other tissues together. In addition it helps with a variety of other functions, including forming and repairing red blood cells, bones, and other tissue; protecting you from bruising by keeping capillary walls and blood vessels firm; keeping your gums healthy; healing cuts and wounds; and keeping your immune system strong and healthy. Vitamin C also helps your body absorb iron from plant sources, which is not as easily absorbed as iron from animals. Vitamin C is one of the very powerful antioxidants that attacks free radicals (unstable molecules with a missing electron formed when the body's cells burn oxygen) in the body's fluids. These free radicals can damage the body's cells, tissues, and even DNA (your body's master plan for reproducing cells).

With pregnancy, a woman's need for vitamin C increases slightly, from 75 mg to 85 mg (for women nineteen to fifty years). Because vitamin C is so readily available in numerous food sources like papayas, bell peppers, pineapple, broccoli, kiwis, cantaloupe, kale, oranges, and strawberries, it is not difficult to get the extra you need.

Minerals

Minerals are also micronutrients. As with vitamins, your good health and your healthy pregnancy require an optimal supply. Minerals do not supply energy to the body directly, because they do not contain calories, but they do fulfill many vital functions. Minerals are part of a baby's bones and teeth. Along with protein and certain vitamins, minerals help to produce blood cells and other body tissues. Minerals aid in numerous body functions that support a normal pregnancy.

Minerals are categorized as either major minerals or trace minerals. Though they are all important, trace minerals are needed in smaller amounts than major minerals. Minerals are absorbed into your intestines and then are transported and stored in your body in various ways. Some minerals pass directly into your bloodstream. They are then transported to the cells, and the excess passes out of the body through the urine. Again, the rule of moderation is the best policy. Although all minerals are important during pregnancy and you should concentrate on getting enough of all of them, some deserve special attention.

Calcium

You already know how vital calcium is to strong bones and teeth. You also know that if your growing baby can't get what she needs, the fetal development process will rob your calcium stores. You need enough calcium to protect your stores and for the development of the baby's bones. Consuming enough calcium during pregnancy may also reduce your chances of developing high blood pressure and toxemia. Calcium requirements do not change throughout pregnancy, but many women still don't consume enough. Regardless of whether you are pregnant, you should consume at least 1,000 mg per day (for women aged nineteen to fifty years). If you do not consume enough calcium-containing foods, such as dairy products, speak to your doctor about calcium supplements. Keep in mind that the upper limit for calcium intake during pregnancy is 2,500 mg per day; this limit will keep you safe from "hypercalcemia," a condition resulting from excessive calcium intake that can lead to unnecessary calcium accumulation in cells (other than bone) that can result in soft tissue calcification.

Iron

As your blood volume increases during the time you are pregnant, your iron needs increase as well. Iron is essential for making hemoglobin, the component of blood that carries oxygen throughout the body and to the baby. Foods rich in vitamin C can help iron be absorbed into the blood. Many women start their pregnancies with less than optimal stores of iron, which can increase their risk of becoming anemic. Women who have iron deficiency anemia may be prescribed a higher dose of iron supplements. You should never increase your iron intake, especially through supplements, without first speaking with your doctor. Iron toxemia, otherwise known as "iron poisoning," is the condition that results from excessive iron intake (most commonly associated with the supplement variety) and can cause symptoms like nausea and vomiting, but also more serious conditions like shock, liver failure, and damage to the lining of the intestinal tract. You can easily avoid any of these possible consequences by simply consulting with your physician prior to taking any kind of iron supplements.

ESSENTIAL

Women who are having multiple babies have slightly higher recommended intakes for some vitamins and minerals. Your doctor can advise you as to your recommended nutritional intake.

Zinc

Almost every cell in the body contains zinc, which is also part of over seventy different types of enzymes. Zinc is known as the second most abundant trace mineral in the human body. Your requirement for this mineral increases slightly during pregnancy from 8 to 11 mg (for women nineteen to fifty years). Zinc is needed for cell growth and brain development. Too much iron from supplements can inhibit the absorption of zinc. Rather than supplementation, you can always opt to include high-zinc foods like oats, yogurt, sesame seeds, pumpkin seeds, and turkey in your diet on a regular basis.

Sodium

Although sodium sometimes gets bad press, it is still a mineral that is essential to life and to good health—and that is still true during pregnancy. Sodium has many important functions in the body, such as controlling the flow of fluids in and out of each cell, regulating blood pressure, transmitting nerve impulses, and helping your muscles relax (including the heart, which is a muscle). Sodium, chloride, and potassium are known as electrolytes, compounds that transmit electrical currents through the body. As a result of these currents, nerve impulses can also be transmitted.

ALERT

Fluid retention, or edema, is very normal during pregnancy and is not always the result of eating too much sodium. Instead, this condition is usually the result of increased estrogen production and a greater blood volume. Do not decrease your sodium intake to relieve edema. Restricting sodium too much can disrupt the body's fluid balance. Extra fluids, especially water, can help relieve some edema. If you are experiencing excessive edema, see your doctor before making any dietary changes.

The terms "salt" and "sodium" are often used interchangeably, yet they are two different things. Sodium is an element of table salt, which is technically known as sodium chloride. How much sodium is in table salt? A single teaspoon of salt contains 2,000 mg of sodium. Generally, articles and guidelines that warn of the dangers of eating too much salt are concerned with sodium only.

Although pregnant women should not decrease their sodium intake, excessive intake is not recommended either. During pregnancy, your body's need for sodium increases. Most women get plenty of sodium in their regular diets, and it is almost never necessary to arrange for extra sodium. In fact, the typical American consumes 4,000 to 8,000 mg per day, well above daily recommended levels. The moderate goal for adults, including pregnant and breastfeeding women, is approximately 2,400 mg of sodium per day.

In healthy people, the kidneys help regulate the sodium level in the body. Sodium levels usually don't become too high because most excess sodium is excreted from the body in urine and through perspiration. For example, when you eat foods that are high in salt, you probably urinate more frequently because the body is trying to rid itself of the extra sodium. Even though your sodium intake may vary from day to day, your body is very efficient at maintaining a proper balance.

Protein

Protein is a powerful macronutrient. During pregnancy, protein provides the material needed for the physical growth and cellular development of the growing baby. Protein is also needed to build the mother's placenta, amniotic tissue, and other maternal tissues. A woman's blood volume increases by almost 50 percent during pregnancy, and additional protein is needed to produce those new blood cells.

FACT

A low protein intake during pregnancy can increase the risk of having a low birth-weight baby. These babies are more prone to health problems and learning disabilities later in life.

During your pregnancy, you need slightly more protein than you did before, and during breastfeeding your needs will continue to increase. The body does not store protein, so you must consume a continuous supply. You need about 10 extra grams of protein from your extra daily calories, or 60 grams of protein daily, compared with the 50 grams a nonpregnant woman requires. Women expecting multiple babies may need more. Here are some examples of where you might find an extra 10 grams of protein:

- In a 1.5-ounce serving of lean meat
- In about 10 ounces of fat-free milk
- In 1.5 ounces of canned tuna in water

Most women do not have a problem meeting their protein requirements. Eating plenty of lean meat, fish, eggs, legumes, and dried beans as well as increasing your dairy servings will ensure you meet your protein needs. If you are a vegetarian and consume plenty of legumes, grain products, soy foods, and vegetables and fruits like summer squashes, cauliflower, collard greens, black beans, split peas, kidney beans, pinto beans, garbanzo beans, and crimini mushrooms, you should not have a problem consuming the recommended amount of protein.

Carbohydrates

You can count on carbohydrates to be your body's main source of energy, especially for the brain and nervous system. Carbohydrates quickly and efficiently convert to energy for mom and baby. Carbohydrates are found in fruits, vegetables, dairy products, starches, and foods in the meat group such as beans and soy products. The only foods in which they are not found are meat, poultry, and fish. Fiber is also considered a carbohydrate and is important to health. However, fiber is not considered a nutrient because most of it is not digested or absorbed into the body.

Good Carbs and Not-So-Good Carbs

Carbohydrates are classified into two different categories: simple carbohydrates, or sugars, and complex carbohydrates, or starches. Sugars are carbohydrates in their simplest form. Refined sugars are found in foods such as table sugar, honey, jams, candy, syrup, and soft drinks. Refined sugars provide calories, but they lack nutrients like vitamins and minerals, and fiber. Some simple sugars, such as those that occur naturally, are found in more nutritious foods, such as the fructose found in fruit or the lactose that is part of dairy products. Complex carbohydrates are basically formed of many simple sugars linked together. They are found in foods such as grains, pasta, rice, vegetables, breads, legumes, nuts, and seeds. Complex carbohydrates are much more nutrient-rich than simple sugars.

How Many Carbs?

On average, women should get approximately 45 to 65 percent of their calories from carbohydrates. Since pregnancy increases calorie needs, more calories must be ingested from carbohydrates. The key is to increase your calories by eating more complex carbohydrates and not more sugar. Take in more complex carbohydrates by eating more fruits and vegetables, whole grains, rice, breads, and cereals. Try adding more beans, lentils, and peas to your daily meals.

FACT

Before complex or simple carbohydrates can be used as energy, they must be broken down into glucose, or blood sugar. Glucose is carried through your bloodstream to your body's cells, where it is converted to energy. Since simple carbohydrates or sugars are already in their simplest form, they go straight into the bloodstream. Complex carbohydrates must be broken down into glucose. Some glucose is used as energy, and some is stored. The hormone insulin helps to regulate your blood sugar.

Following the USDA's MyPlate guidelines and eating the suggested number of servings from each food group during pregnancy will give you a safe suggested guideline that you are consuming the amount of carbohydrates your body needs for a healthy pregnancy and a healthy baby. Even though carbohydrates are extremely important, they need to be balanced with the other two macronutrients: protein and fat.

Fat

Fat is an important nutrient that sometimes gets a bad rap. Its major functions in the body include providing an energy source, aiding in the absorption and transport of the fat-soluble vitamins A, D, E, and K, cushioning organs, and regulating body temperature. All women, pregnant or not, should get 20 to 35 percent of their calories from fat. Fat can be dangerous to health if consumed in excess or if the wrong kinds of fat are eaten. It is important to include fat in your daily diet but in moderation. Fat is a very concentrated source of calories. A gram of fat has 9 calories, twice as many as a gram of carbohydrates or protein (both of which contain 4 calories per gram). A small amount of fat can go a long way!

Good Fat Versus Bad Fat

There are different types of triglycerides, or dietary fats. Some of these fats are more harmful than others. The major kinds of fats in the foods you eat are saturated, polyunsaturated, monounsaturated, and trans-fatty acids or hydrogenated fats. The unsaturated fats (polyunsaturated and monounsaturated) are referred to as the "healthy" fats. These fats can help to lower cholesterol levels, and they also have heart-protective factors. Most of the fat in your diet should be unsaturated. Following is a list of foods that contain healthy fats:

- Almonds
- Avocado oil
- Bee pollen
- Canola oil
- Cashews
- Coconut oil
- Flaxseeds
- Hemp seeds
- Olive oil
- Pistachios
- Walnuts

Sources of monounsaturated fats include certain plant-based oils, such as olive, canola, and peanut. Avocados are also good sources of monounsaturated fats. Sources of polyunsaturated fats include certain other plant-based oils such as corn, cottonseed, safflower, sunflower, sesame, and soybean. Nuts and seeds are also good sources. This group also includes the omega-3 fatty acids found in some fish. There are two polyunsaturated essential fatty acids that your body does not make and you must get from the food you consume. These two fatty acids are linoleic acid (or omega-6) and linolenic acid (or omega-3).

Saturated fats and trans-fatty acids tend to increase blood cholesterol levels, which can lead to health problems such as heart disease and stroke. The major sources of saturated fat are animal foods such as meat, poultry, and whole-milk dairy products. However, some plant sources also provide saturated fat, including palm and palm kernel oils. Food that contains trans-fats includes some margarines, cookies, crackers, and other commercial baked goods made with partially hydrogenated vegetable oils, as well as French fries, donuts, and other commercial fried foods.

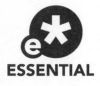

ESSENTIAL

Eating a totally fat-free diet is not part of a healthy eating style. Fat is an essential nutrient, and some fats—such as omega-3 fatty acids—are necessary for certain parts of a baby's development. A totally fat-free diet may also fail to provide sufficient calories.

Trimming the Fat

Fat is definitely a needed nutrient in a healthy diet. The problem is that most Americans consume too much and the wrong kinds. Don't cut fat completely out of your diet, but it is important to cut back and to choose the right types. This means lowering your intake of dietary cholesterol and saturated fat. You should also lower your blood cholesterol or maintain it at safe levels as a way of decreasing your risk for heart disease.

FACT

Cholesterol is not the same as fat. Cholesterol is a fat-like substance, but it has a different structure and different functions in the body than fat does. Because cholesterol provides no energy to the body, it has no calories.

You can cut the fat and cholesterol from your meals without losing any flavor. For example, try using egg whites or egg substitute in place of whole eggs. Choose leaner meats, cook with skinless poultry and fish, or occasionally opt for a vegetarian meal with beans or soy products as your main protein source. Read the nutrition facts panel to keep an eye on your daily intake of total fat, saturated fat, and cholesterol.

Fiber

Fiber is exclusively found in plant foods; it is the part of the plant that your body cannot digest. Fiber, also called dietary fiber, is categorized as a complex carbohydrate, but because it cannot be digested or absorbed into your bloodstream, it is not considered a nutrient. There are two types of fiber: soluble and insoluble. Each type has a different beneficial health function in the body. It is important to eat a variety of fiber-rich foods every day that will provide you with the health benefits of both soluble and insoluble fiber.

Soluble Fibers

Soluble fibers naturally found in plants include gums, mucilages, psyllium, and pectins. Foods that contain these fibers include peas, beans, oats, barley, and some fruits (especially apples with skin, oranges, prunes, strawberries, and bananas) and some vegetables (especially carrots, broccoli, and cauliflower). Soluble fiber binds to fatty substances and promotes their excretion, which in turn seems to help lower blood cholesterol levels.

FACT

According to the American Heart Association, soluble fibers, when part of your everyday low-fat and low-cholesterol diet, can aid in slowing the absorption of sugar into the bloodstream, which in turn can help to control your blood sugar levels.

Insoluble Fibers

Insoluble fiber is known as "roughage." The insoluble fibers give plants their structure. Insoluble fibers naturally found in plants include cellulose, hemicellulose, and lignin. Foods that contain these fibers include whole-wheat or whole-grain products, wheat bran, corn bran, some fruits (especially the skin), and many vegetables including cauliflower, green beans, potatoes with skin, and broccoli. Insoluble fibers do not dissolve in water, but they hold on to water as they move waste through your intestinal tract. By holding on to water, they add bulk and softness to the stool and therefore promote regularity and help prevent constipation. Insoluble fibers also help accelerate intestinal transit time, which means they decrease the amount of time that waste stays in the colon. This cuts the time that potentially harmful waste food substances can linger in the intestines.

Fiber Benefits

Basically, fiber comes in and goes out of the body. However, it does some pretty amazing things on its travels. Fiber helps to promote good health in many ways. Studies show that a diet rich in fiber as part of a varied, balanced, and low-fat eating pattern may help to prevent some chronic diseases. No matter how good your present health is you can certainly benefit from adding more fiber to your diet. Fiber not only promotes health but also may help to reduce the risk for digestive problems, heart disease, some types of cancer, and diabetes. A fiber-rich diet can also help to promote weight management.

ALERT

There is such a thing as too much of a good thing. Eating more than 50 to 60 grams of fiber per day may cause a decrease in the amount of vitamins and minerals, such as zinc, iron, magnesium, and calcium, that your body absorbs. Large amounts of fiber can also cause gas, diarrhea, and bloating.

How Much Is Enough?

A diet rich in fiber is important at all times, but it can be especially helpful during pregnancy. A fiber-rich diet can help to prevent constipation, which plagues many pregnant women. The average American only eats about 12 to 17 grams of fiber daily, which is well below the recommended levels, so make sure you make the necessary changes to your diet to boost your fiber! Adults under the age of fifty should get 25 grams a day; adults over fifty should get 21 grams. When boosting your fiber intake, it is important to increase your intake gradually and to make sure you are drinking plenty of fluids.

Adding fiber to your diet may be easier than you think. Just looking at the fiber content on the nutrition facts panel on packaged foods can help you be aware of what you need to do to increase your fiber intake. Choose foods that are good sources of fiber and have at least 2.5 grams or more of fiber per serving. Make simple switches by substituting higher-fiber foods, such as whole-grain breads, brown rice, whole-wheat pasta, fruits, and vegetables for lower-fiber foods such as white bread, white rice, candy, and chips. Eat more raw vegetables and fresh fruits, and include the skins when appropriate. Lightly steam these foods, which can preserve a lot of the fiber content. Plan your meals to include high-fiber foods such as fruits, vegetables, legumes, or whole-grain starches. Simply adding extra vegetables to your favorite sandwiches, soups, and casseroles can make a world of difference.

ESSENTIAL

Don't consider juice for daily servings of fruit! Whole fruits contain more fiber than juice because much of the fiber is found in the skin and pulp, which is removed when the juice is made.

What better way to start your day than with a high-fiber breakfast cereal such as bran cereal or oatmeal? Look for cereals that contain at least 3 to 5 grams or more of fiber per serving. Add some fresh fruit to the top of your cereal for an extra fiber boost. Since both soluble and insoluble fibers are important for good health, eat a variety of high-fiber foods to ensure you get a mix of both types of fiber. Make good use of your snacks by choosing those that will increase your fiber intake. Nibble on dried fruits, popcorn, fresh fruit, raw vegetables, whole-wheat bagels, or whole-wheat crackers. Try something different and add legumes, or dried beans, to your diet at least two to three times per week. You can add them to salads, soups, casseroles, or spaghetti sauce.

Phytochemicals

Phytochemicals, also known as phytonutrients, are compounds found naturally in plant-based foods—such as fruits, vegetables, legumes, whole grains, nuts, and seeds—that may provide potential health benefits. Phytonutrients are compounds that plants provide naturally to protect themselves against things like viruses, bacteria, and fungi. These phytonutrients are on the cutting edge of health-promoting potential. Though their role is still uncertain, particular phytonutrients may help protect against illnesses including heart disease, certain cancers, high blood pressure, osteoporosis, stroke, cataracts, and other chronic health conditions. There are thousands of phytonutrients—you could find more than 2,000 in the pigments that give plants their color. The more colorful your produce, the more phytonutrients it contains.

CHAPTER 5

Best (and Worst!) Foods for Pregnancy

Even with the best intentions to eat healthier foods, max out nutrition, and steer clear of the foods that are void of nutrition (or downright dangerous!), it can be a little overwhelming to find out the best foods for pregnancy. From your favorite fruits and vegetables to the perfect proteins and gracious grains that can make your pregnancy a delightfully delicious and nutritious one . . . with the added element of safety, knowing the best foods from which to choose can make pregnant life a little easier.

Fruits

Sweet, juicy, and satisfying, the plentiful phytochemical-packed fruits that top the nutrition charts for pregnancy offer enough variety that you can surely find some you like. Satisfying your sweet tooth with a crisp apple or juicy kiwi can help curb cravings for unhealthy alternatives, and offer up the perfect snack-sized option that's the perfect on-the-go energy-boosting treat! Here are some examples of fabulous fruits you can add to your healthy diet:

- Apples
- Avocado
- Bananas
- Blackberries
- Blueberries
- Cantaloupe
- Grapefruit
- Grapes
- Honeydew melons
- Kiwi
- Lemons
- Limes
- Mango
- Oranges
- Papayas
- Peaches
- Pears
- Pineapple
- Pomegranates
- Raspberries
- Strawberries
- Tomatoes

One of the best tricks to keep your fruit intake on track is to keep your favorite fruit choices in your fridge and on your countertop. If you find yourself looking for a snack or meal and can't decide what would satisfy your hunger, a long stare in the fridge that's packed with an assortment of beautiful and delicious fruit is, more often than not, going to result in a healthy choice that will satisfy your hunger, your sweet tooth, *and* suggested fruit servings.

Vegetables

If you find yourself in a recipe rut, or don't know much about veggie options available, find comfort in knowing that the choices for fresh veggies are so numerous that you could try a new variety every day for weeks until you find the ones you love! Packed with plentiful vitamins, minerals, and phytochemicals, adding colorful veggies to every meal is a must . . . and a nutritious plus in pregnancy. Try these vibrant vegetables:

- Beets
- Broccoli
- Cabbage
- Carrots
- Cauliflower
- Celery
- Corn
- Green beans
- Kale

- Onions
- Peas
- Peppers
- Potatoes
- Romaine lettuce
- Spinach
- Squash
- Sweet potatoes
- Zucchini

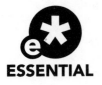

ESSENTIAL

If you're going to spend the time and money to stock your fridge with fresh vegetables, you can make it easier to use them up by prepping them ahead. Rather than letting vegetables go bad because you feel like it will take forever to prep them, chop, dice, and slice the vegetables within twenty-four to forty-eight hours after bringing them home. You'll save money, save time, and save the guilt of wasting precious foods.

Protein

Meats, poultry, fish, dry beans, eggs, nuts, and dairy are sources of protein. This group supplies large amounts of protein as well as other essential nutrients including zinc, iron, B vitamins, and calcium. Meats can also be a large source of saturated fat and cholesterol, so it is important to choose lean cuts.

With seafood, meat, or poultry, look for labels marked "lean." This means that each 3-ounce serving includes the following:

- Less than 10 grams of total fat
- 4 grams of saturated fat
- 95 mg cholesterol

For products marked "extra lean," a 3-ounce serving includes:

- Less than 5 grams total fat
- 2 grams saturated fat
- 95 mg cholesterol

ALERT

Although soy can be a healthy alternative to animal foods, recent studies done on animals found that certain soy components consumed during pregnancy may adversely affect the sexual development of male offspring. Even though no affects have been observed in Asia, where soy is a major part of the diet, the studies have sparked concern and warrant further studies. If you are vegetarian, try not to rely solely on soy for your main source of protein but choose other foods for variety.

Lean Beef and Pork

Protein foods that come from animal sources can be confusing when it comes to fat content, so it is important to choose wisely. Choose leaner cuts of beef, which you can usually tell by their names: "round" cuts, such as eye of round or round roast, or "loin" cuts, such as tenderloin or sirloin. Other lean cuts include the flank (such as flank steak), porterhouse steak or roast, and T-bone steak. For leaner cuts of pork, choose a name that includes "loin," such as loin chop or tenderloin.

Always buy meat that is well trimmed, with no more than an eighth of an inch of visible fat trim. Trim refers to the fat layer surrounding the cut of meat. Marbled fat is the fat within the meat that shows as white streaks throughout the piece of meat. Marbled fat can't be trimmed, but with the correct cooking methods like grilling or using certain drip pans that allow excess fat to fall away from the meat, it can be somewhat decreased. Check packages of meat to find the highest lean-to-fat ratio.

When it comes to ground beef, choose leaner varieties. Ground beef that is 95 percent lean meets government standards for "lean." Ground round is the leanest ground beef, followed by ground sirloin, ground chuck, and regular ground meat.

Ensure that meat is fresh by checking out the color. Beef is typically bright red, young veal and pork are grayish-pink, and older veal is a darker pink. Check the dates on meat also because with some meat items, such as ground beef, exposure to oxygen, even under plastic wrap, can cause the outer layer of the meat to darken.

Poultry

Poultry is a bit leaner than some red meats, but it is still important to know some essential tips. Choose leaner varieties of poultry such as chicken and turkey, and choose skinless to make it easier to trim fat before cooking. If buying poultry with skin, remove the skin before cooking. Try ground turkey for a leaner alternative to ground beef. Be sure the ground turkey package states "lean" or "very lean," which means it is made from white-meat turkey. The fat content is higher if it is ground with dark meat and skin.

If you're buying a whole turkey, keep in mind that self-basting varieties are usually higher in fat because they are injected with fat to help preserve moisture. For freshness, check dates and look for meaty poultry with skin that is creamy white to yellow and that is free of bruises, tiny feathers, and torn or dry skin. Also check the nutrition facts panel. Some of these foods may not be as low in fat as you assume, and some may be high in sodium.

Fish

Fish can be a wonderful source of some very healthy fats. Most fish has less fat than meat or poultry, and most of the fat from fish is a polyunsaturated source (a healthy fat) such as omega-3 fatty acid. Fattier fish has more omega-3 fatty acids than lean fish or shellfish, and these fats may offer heart-healthy benefits. Fish that is white or light in color, such as perch, orange roughy, snapper, and sole, is lower in fat than fish that is firm and darker in color, such as mackerel and salmon. Always check the dates on fish to make sure it is fresh, and for safety do not buy cooked seafood that is displayed alongside raw fish or seafood.

Fish and seafood can be a valuable source of nutrition. Fish contains protein, omega-3 fatty acids, vitamin D, and other essential nutrients that make it an exceptionally healthy food for pregnant mothers and developing babies. However, some fish can contain harmful levels of methyl mercury, a toxic mercury compound. Mercury occurs naturally in the environment and is often released into the air through industrial pollution. From the air, mercury can fall and accumulate in streams, lakes, and oceans where fish is caught for consumption. Bacteria in the water can cause chemical changes that transform mercury into the toxic form of methyl mercury. Fish in these bodies of water absorb methyl mercury as they feed on organisms within the water.

QUESTION

Can I eat tuna salad while pregnant?
Guidelines released by the EPA (Environmental Protection Agency) and the FDA (Food and Drug Administration) in March 2004 state that albacore tuna ("white tuna") as well as tuna steaks have higher mercury levels than canned light tuna. You can eat up to 6 ounces (one average meal) of albacore tuna per week. Even if you choose to use the canned light tuna, it is best to eat only one average meal of the tuna and choose another meal from another type of fish since the new advisory also suggests eating a variety of fish every week.

If consumed regularly by women who can become pregnant, women who are pregnant or nursing, or by a young child, methyl mercury can harm a developing brain and nervous system. Just about all types of fish contain trace amounts of methyl mercury, which is not harmful to most humans. However, larger fish that feed on other fish accumulate the highest levels of methyl mercury. These types of fish pose the greatest risks to people that consume them on a regular basis. Any risk comes from a buildup of mercury in the body and not from a single meal. The FDA and EPA advise women who are pregnant or could become pregnant, nursing mothers, and young children not to eat shark, swordfish, king mackerel, or tilefish because these fish contain higher, unsafe levels of methyl mercury.

ALERT

If you follow a strict vegan diet, you still need to ensure that you consume plenty of protein as well as the other nutrients that this food group supplies. Your doctor may prescribe additional supplements, and a dietitian can help you devise a well-balanced eating plan.

It is smart to keep abreast of guidelines concerning the consumption of fish during pregnancy. Many organizations are trying to enforce stricter guidelines than are currently being recommended by the FDA and EPA. Check out the EPA website at *www.epa.gov* and the FDA website at *www .fda.gov* for the latest advisories.

Dairy

The dairy group includes milk, yogurt, cheese, cottage cheese, and even favorites such as ice cream and frozen yogurt. Because they are an animal source, dairy foods can also contribute to saturated fat and cholesterol intake, so choosing lower-fat or fat-free versions of these foods can help keep your levels down.

To make sure you get the nutrients you need without too many calories and saturated fat, choose low-fat or fat-free milk, yogurt, cheese, and cottage cheese. Low-fat cheese has 3 grams or less of fat per serving. Cheeses that are made with low-fat milk are also lower in fat, such as part-skim mozzarella. Yogurt is a wonderful food, but fruited yogurts tend to range widely in calorie and fat content, so it is important to check the nutrition facts panel. For optimal freshness, look for the sell-by date (the last date on which the food should be sold) on dairy foods. If lactose intolerance is a problem for you, look for lactose-reduced or lactose-free milk and other dairy products. Soy milk is lactose free, but make sure the brand you choose is fortified with calcium.

FACT

Cottage cheese has less calcium than other dairy products because during processing, the whey, which contains 50 to 75 percent of the calcium, is drained away. Look for cottage cheese products that are processed with extra calcium. Cottage cheese still contains plenty of protein and riboflavin and little fat.

Other Protein Options

Eggs are a good source of protein. Egg yolks contain a significant amount of fat and cholesterol. The refrigerated egg substitutes available at your grocery store offer a cholesterol-free and lower-fat option. Always check the expiration date on eggs for freshness.

Some plant-based foods, including dried beans, peas, and lentils, are excellent sources of protein and fiber. Choose these as an alternative to meat a few times a week and add them to salads, casseroles, soups, or stews. Soy products such as tofu, soy milk, and veggie burgers can also be an excellent source of protein, and they make a good alternative to meat occasionally. They are low in fat, contain no cholesterol, and are good sources of fiber.

Grains

Whole grains are an important source of the complex carbohydrates that are a major source of energy for both you and the baby. Breads, cereals, rice, and pasta should make up the base of your diet. Grain foods also supply vitamin E, B vitamins such as folic acid, and minerals such as magnesium, iron, and zinc. Whole grains are also rich in fiber.

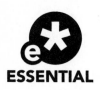

ESSENTIAL

Whole grains are much more nutritious than refined grains. Refined grains, such as white bread, go through a process that strips them of nutritious parts of the grain. Nutrients such as thiamin, riboflavin, niacin, and folic acid are lost. In some cases the lost nutrients are added back to the product, which is advertised as "enriched." Foods may also be labeled as "fortified," which means that nutrients have been added that were not originally found in the food.

Here are some examples of foods that provide whole grains to your diet:

- Bran cereal
- Rolled oats
- Cream of wheat
- Buckwheat
- 100% whole-wheat bread
- Sprouted-grain bread
- 100% whole-wheat pasta

- 100% whole-wheat tortillas
- Bulgur
- Quinoa
- Millet
- Wheat germ

When buying bread, read the label to check that whole-wheat flour is the first ingredient listed. If the label specifies whole wheat or whole grain, the bread also contains fiber. Look for bread that provides at least 2 grams of fiber per slice. If you are not a fan of whole-wheat breads, keep in mind that other breads contain fiber, including rye and pumpernickel. Try different brands of whole-wheat bread to find one that you enjoy. When you are shopping for your grain products, look for labels that read "high in fiber" or "good source of fiber." Choose grain or starch products made with little or no fat and less sugar. In other words, instead of the croissant, go for the whole-wheat bagel. Take advantage of the fiber that cereals can provide. Choose cereals that offer at least 3 grams of fiber, have 3 grams of fat or less, and include 8 grams or less of sugar per serving.

QUESTION

Are all wheat breads the same?
Just because bread is labeled "wheat" or "multigrain" or because it is brown in color does not necessarily mean it is high in fiber or even that it has fiber at all. In some breads, the brown color comes from caramel coloring, which must be included in the ingredient list. By law, bread labeled "whole wheat" must be made from 100 percent whole-wheat flour. Bread labeled simply as "wheat" can include both wheat and refined white flour, and proportions vary from product to product.

Don't leave out cooked cereal such as oatmeal, grits, or cream of wheat that can be low in fat and high in fiber. Making simple changes, like choosing brown rice over white rice, can pack in a lot more nutrition and fiber. Brown rice is the only type of whole-grain rice, and it contains more fiber and B vitamins than white rice. Whole-wheat or whole-grain pasta is higher in fiber and B vitamins than regular pasta. Experiment with other grains such as quinoa, millet, or couscous. Get in the habit of looking for the word "whole" in front of grains such as barley, corn, oats, rice, or wheat. Always check the expiration dates on your grain products for freshness. Lastly, keep an eye on various breads like dinner rolls, sandwich bread, or buns—these can pack in the calories unless you pay attention. Check labels for calories per serving.

Sugars

In moderation, sugar can be part of a healthy diet. Sugar belongs to the carbohydrate group, which also includes starches and fibers. Natural sugars are found in fruit (in the form of fructose) and milk (as lactose). Sugar becomes a dietary culprit when it is added to other foods (usually processed items). Major sources of added sugar are those found in soft drinks, candy, pastries, cookies, ice cream, and other sweets. Although the body does not know the difference between sugar and complex carbohydrates, most sugars are referred to as "empty calories" because they provide calories but very little or no nutritional value. Satisfy your sweet tooth, but do it in moderation.

What's Okay to Eat?

The typical American diet is packed with too much sugar, and nutrition experts agree that Americans need to cut back. The idea behind a healthy pregnancy diet is to eat foods that really count toward your nutritional intake. Eating too many sugary foods means lots of extra calories and very little nutrition. Eating too many of these foods also tends to bump out the more nutritious foods that you should be choosing. Foods with lots of added sugar should only be occasional treats, not regular snacks.

Though there is no established recommended daily allowance (RDA) for sugar, you should concentrate on getting the bulk of your carbohydrates from complex sources—such as breads, rice, and pasta—and most of your simple carbohydrates from fruits and dairy products, which also contain vitamins, minerals, and fiber.

Read Food Labels

The FDA requires sugar content to be included on all nutrition facts panels. The panel lists total carbohydrates and sugar in terms of grams per serving. Sugar is part of the total carbohydrate amount that is listed. If you purchase a food with added sugar, make sure it also provides plenty of nutrients such as vitamins and minerals, and fiber.

ALERT

When checking the ingredient labels on packaged food, you will find all types of sweeteners listed. The suffix "-ose" (fructose, sucrose, lactose) indicates that an ingredient is a form of sugar. Look for these other ingredients that indicate added sugar: brown sugar, corn sweetener, corn syrup, fruit juice concentrate, high-fructose corn syrup, honey, invert sugar, lactose, molasses, and raw sugar.

Foods to Avoid

Although the food supply in the Unites States is one of the safest in the world, the way you store, prepare, and/or handle food after it leaves the grocery store can put you at risk for food-borne illness or food poisoning. Some foods can carry harmful bacteria and parasites that can make both you and your baby sick. Pregnant women are in the higher-risk category when it comes to contracting food-borne bacteria, such as salmonella, staphylococcus aureus, E. coli, clostridium perfringens, toxoplasma gondii, or listeria monocytogenes. Some food-borne bacteria can be more harmful to the mother and baby than others.

Symptoms of Food-Borne Illness

Symptoms of food-borne illnesses can develop as soon as thirty minutes or as much as three weeks after a contaminated food is eaten. Since symptoms can mimic those of the flu, it is important to know the differences. If you have flu-like symptoms but they don't go away within twenty-four to forty-eight hours, that could be a sign of something more serious, such as food-borne illness. If you vomit, have diarrhea more than two times per day, have bloody diarrhea, have a stiff neck with a severe headache and fever, or if your symptoms last for more than three days, you should call your doctor immediately. If your doctor suspects a food-borne illness, he can perform a blood antibody test for certain bacteria or parasites.

ALERT

Toxoplasma gondii, or T. gondii, is a parasitic infection that can contaminate food. This parasite can result in toxoplasmosis, which usually causes mild to no symptoms for pregnant women; but there is a 40 percent chance that it can be passed to the developing fetus. T. gondii can cause miscarriage and disability. Most often, it is contracted from eating undercooked meat and poultry or unwashed fruits and vegetables, from contamination of cleaning a cat's litter box, or from handling contaminated soil.

Listeria Monocytogenes

Listeria monocytogenes is a bacteria on some foods that can cause a serious infection, called listeriosis, in humans. Most people who eat listeria-contaminated foods do not get ill. However, pregnant women are twenty times more likely than other healthy adults to get listeriosis and become seriously ill. Listeriosis results in an estimated 2,500 serious illnesses and 500 deaths each year.

Pregnant women, older adults, and people with weakened immune systems are at higher risk for contracting listeriosis. This food-borne illness can cause the most serious harm to a fetus, resulting in miscarriages, fetal death, severe illness, and even the death of a newborn. If a person has three telltale symptoms—stiff neck, severe headache, and fever—she may have listeria.

Listeria monocytogenes can grow at refrigerator temperatures and can be found in ready-to-eat foods. Listeria can also contaminate other foods, and contaminated foods may not look, smell, or even taste any different than uncontaminated foods. Eat perishable foods that are precooked or ready-to-eat as soon as possible. Clean your refrigerator on a regular basis, and keep a thermometer in your refrigerator to make sure it stays at 40°F or below. These steps can help reduce your risk for listeriosis as well as other food-borne illnesses. Thorough cooking at the correct temperatures can kill the listeria bacteria.

Some foods have a greater likelihood of containing listeria monocytogenes and can put you at greater risk for other food-borne illnesses. Pregnant women should *completely avoid* the following foods:

- Hot dogs and luncheon meats, unless they are reheated until steaming hot (at least 165°F)
- Soft cheeses such as feta, goat cheese, Brie, Camembert, blue-veined cheeses such as Roquefort, and Mexican-style soft cheeses such as queso blanco fresco. It is acceptable to eat hard cheese such as Cheddar; semi-soft cheese such as mozzarella; pasteurized processed cheese such as slices and spreads; cream cheeses; and cottage cheese
- Pâtés and/or meat spreads. It is acceptable to eat canned or shelf-stable pâtés and meat spreads
- Refrigerated smoked seafood, unless contained in a cooked dish such as a casserole
- Raw (unpasteurized) milk or foods that contain unpasteurized milk
- Unpasteurized juices and ciders
- Raw sprouts
- Dishes including raw or undercooked eggs including eggnog, cake batter, raw cookie dough, some Caesar salad dressings, and hollandaise sauce
- Raw or undercooked shellfish or seafood, including sushi
- Undercooked meats, poultry, and eggs

CHAPTER 6

The Vegetarian or Vegan Mom-to-Be

Becoming a vegetarian is an important step for many women, usually fueled by a desire to create optimal changes within the self or for the world. Regardless of the type of vegetarian you are, it is completely safe to remain vegetarian throughout pregnancy. Although many decades of speculation have led people to consider vegetarianism inadequate in certain nutrients like protein, B_{12}, iron, and other vitamins and minerals, studies have shown that a well-planned vegetarian diet can include more than enough of the essential nutrients needed. During pregnancy, including a variety of highly nutritious foods providing bountiful protein, omega-3s, and vitamins and minerals will ensure the health of mom and baby from conception to delivery and beyond.

Is a Vegetarian Diet Safe During Pregnancy?

Regardless of the vegetarian category you choose for your lifestyle, you and your baby will not only benefit from the foods you consume, you can thrive! By focusing on including a wide variety of natural foods in your diet, you can keep your diet cleaner and healthier than most with the added benefit of naturally occurring phytochemicals that have been shown to safeguard health and promote healthy development. While a pregnant diet will require a little extra persistence, focus, and planning, a vegetarian mom-to-be can remain vegetarian throughout pregnancy by being aware of the types of foods included in every meal to ensure that no specific foods such as greens or grains are being excluded or consumed on a minimal basis. Each fruit, vegetable, seed, grain, nut, and legume provides a very different combination of macro- and micronutrients, so a deficiency in one food group would likely result in a deficiency in the diet and, eventually, within the body.

A healthy vegetarian pregnancy diet must be balanced. In other words, it must contain all of the nutrients essential to good health and a healthy pregnancy. It may take a little work, but keep in mind that knowledge is power. The more you know about the foods you eat, the more nutritious your diet can become. The nutritional adequacy of a vegetarian diet depends more on the overall food choices made over several days than what you consume at each meal.

The Benefits

Vegetarian diets can be very healthy if designed correctly. A healthy, well-planned vegetarian diet usually contains more fiber. It is also lower in total fat, especially saturated fat and dietary cholesterol, which can help lower the risk for diseases such as heart disease, stroke, and some cancers. In addition, LDL blood cholesterol (the "bad" cholesterol) levels are generally lower in vegetarians, which can decrease the incidence of death from heart disease. Vegetarians tend to have a lower incidence of hypertension, type 2 diabetes, obesity, and some forms of cancers, such as lung and colon, than people who eat meat.

Vegetarian diets that are high in fruits, vegetables, and whole grains also tend to be higher in folic acid, antioxidants such as vitamins C and E, carotenoids, and phytochemicals. All these benefits give this eating style an extra disease-fighting punch. However, the key to being at a lower risk for these health problems is following a properly balanced vegetarian diet.

ESSENTIAL

Keep in mind that not all vegetarian protein sources are low in fat. Popular protein sources, such as nuts and seeds, can be high in fat. These contain unsaturated (or healthy) fats, but small amounts can pack in lots of calories.

The Pitfalls

It is important to keep in mind that being a vegetarian does not guarantee that you are eating a healthy diet. A poorly planned vegetarian diet can cause some nutritional deficiencies. It can also be high in fat, cholesterol, and calories and low in fiber. Some vegetarians may have a high saturated-fat intake from consuming too many eggs, cream, butter, whole-milk products, and cheese. Vegetarians may get into the rut of eating too many low-fiber starches without including enough of the other food groups, such as plant-based proteins, fruits, vegetables, whole grains, and dairy foods (if included in their eating style).

FACT

Vegetarian women who are breastfeeding need to make sure they are consuming plenty of vitamin B_{12} sources because intake can affect levels in breast milk. While you are on prenatal vitamins, you should get all of the nutrients you need. After delivery, your doctor will most likely take you off your prenatal vitamins. Talk to your doctor or a dietitian about starting a multivitamin/mineral supplement that will ensure optimal nutritional intake.

Despite some of the pitfalls of a vegetarian diet, you can still reap the benefits of a vegetarian lifestyle as long as you plan your meals correctly and you eat higher-fat, higher-sugar foods in moderation.

The Vegetarian Food Guide Pyramid

The Vegetarian Food Guide Pyramid is very similar to the regular Food Guide Pyramid. The vegetarian version provides recommended guidelines for the vegetarian population. The lacto-ovo vegetarian diet can be modified to meet the guidelines of the Food Guide Pyramid with only a few modifications. If you consume eggs and/or dairy products, choose lower-fat or nonfat products to limit the amount of saturated fat and cholesterol you consume each day.

The following list describes the minimum number of servings you should consume from each food group during pregnancy:

- **Use fats, oils, and sweets sparingly.** This includes candy, butter, margarine, salad dressing, and cooking oil.
- **Eat three to four servings from the milk, yogurt, and cheese group.** Examples of single servings from this group include 1 cup of milk or yogurt or 1½ ounces of cheese. Those who choose not to eat milk, yogurt, or cheese should select other food sources rich in calcium, such as calcium-fortified juice, cereal, dark-green leafy vegetables, and soy milk.
- **Eat two servings (6–7 ounces each) from the dry beans, nuts, seeds, eggs, and meat substitutes group.** Examples of a single serving from this food group include 1 cup of soy milk, ½ cup of cooked dry beans or peas, one egg or two egg whites, ⅓ cup of nuts or seeds, or 2 tablespoons peanut butter. Shoot to eat at least three to four servings of cooked dried beans weekly. They are a good choice because they are full of zinc, iron, protein, and fiber.
- **Eat four servings from the vegetable group.** Examples of a single serving from this group include ½ cup of cooked or chopped raw vegetables or 1 cup of raw leafy vegetables. Choose dark-green leafy vegetables often for higher calcium intake.
- **Eat three servings from the fruit group.** Examples of a single serving from this group include ¾ cup of juice, ¼ cup of dried fruit, ½ cup of chopped raw fruit, ½ cup of canned fruit, or a medium-size piece of fruit, such as banana, apple, or orange.
- **Eat nine servings from the bread, cereal, rice, and pasta group.** Examples of a single serving from this group include one slice of bread, 1 ounce of ready-to-eat cereal, ½ cup of cooked cereal, ½ cup of cooked

brown rice, pasta, or other grains, or half a bagel. Those consuming gluten should choose whole-wheat and whole-grain breads and pastas more often, as well as fortified and enriched products, while gluten-free diets should include more rice, rice pastas, and gluten-free breads and cereals.

Vegetarian Meal Planning Tips

The key to a healthy vegetarian diet is making the right choices and eating a variety of foods. It never hurts to take an overall look at your diet to make sure it is well balanced, nutritious, and in line with your new pregnancy needs. There are all kinds of specialty foods out there that you may have never thought of trying. Here are a few suggestions to get you started:

- Explore new foods at your grocery store. Instead of going with the same old foods, try new grains (such as barley, bulgur, couscous, kasha, and quinoa), vegetables, and/or legumes each week.
- Try different meat-free or soy products from the selection located in the freezer section or the health section. Soy can boost the protein, calcium, and iron content of almost any meal.
- Add different types of legumes or dried beans to casseroles, stews, soups, salads, and chili for a protein, iron, zinc, and fiber boost to your meal.
- Prepare some of your favorite dishes with a soy substitute, such as using textured vegetable protein in Sloppy Joes or spaghetti sauce or adding cubed tofu to a stir-fry along with your favorite vegetables.
- Next time you grill out, try a marinated portabella mushroom or veggie burger marinated in teriyaki sauce or your favorite marinade.
- Buy a vegetarian cookbook, or search out vegetarian recipes that meet your specific criteria, likes, and dislikes on the Internet for new ideas. The websites *www.vegweb.com*, *www.fatfree.com*, and *www .vegkitchen.com* should get you started.
- When looking for a place to dine out, suggest Chinese, Vietnamese, Thai, or Italian. You can always find plenty of vegetarian entrées on these menus.

ESSENTIAL

If you are a vegan, you may have a tougher time making sure you consume all of the essential nutrients you need during pregnancy. You need to make modifications to the Food Guide Pyramid to fit your lifestyle, but also ensure your nutrient intake is meeting your requirements. Seek the guidance of a dietitian who can make sure you are planning your diet correctly.

Special Vitamin and Mineral Considerations

If you are not careful, eliminating animal foods from your diet can cause a shortfall of several nutrients in an otherwise healthy eating plan. Nutrients that should be given special attention include calcium, vitamin D, iron, vitamin B_{12}, and zinc. You should notify your doctor of your vegetarian eating style so that she is aware of your nutrient intake and can prescribe supplements you might need. In addition, careful meal planning and good choices can ensure the intake of all these essential nutrients each day. Keep in mind that you should never take additional supplements without first speaking to your doctor. It is possible to overdo a good thing! If you have questions about how you can combine foods to incorporate essential vitamins and minerals, speak to a registered dietitian.

Calcium

Calcium is vital for strong bones and teeth for both the baby and the mother. Pregnant women need 1,000 mg per day. For vegetarian moms who consume dairy products (at least three servings of dairy foods each day), consuming enough calcium should not be a problem. For vegans, however, calcium intake can be a concern. However, calcium can be found in both plant and animal foods.

Though it may take a bit more planning, as a pregnant vegan you can definitely find foods that fit your eating style and contain enough calcium to help you meet your daily needs. Some of these foods include tofu processed with calcium, calcium-fortified beverages such as orange juice and soy milk, calcium-fortified breakfast cereals, broccoli, seeds such as sunflower and sesame, tahini, nuts such as almonds, soy beans, legumes, some greens such as kale, mustard greens, and collards, bok choy, okra, dried figs, and almond butter.

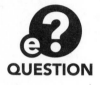

Is it okay to take a calcium supplement if I don't eat dairy foods?
If you can't get enough calcium from the foods you choose, a supplement can be a good idea. The rule of thumb should always be food before supplements, though. First, include calcium-containing foods in your diet as much as possible, and then supplement on top of that. Never let a supplement take the place of an entire food group or nutrient such as calcium.

Vitamin D

Vitamin D is essential to help the body absorb calcium and phosphorus and then deposit them into teeth and bones. Your body can also make vitamin D when your skin is exposed to sunlight. With the exception of milk, very few foods are naturally high in vitamin D. If you are a vegetarian who drinks milk, vitamin D should not be a concern if you consume the recommended number of servings. However, if you are a vegan, you need to be careful that you get enough vitamin D in your diet. The best way for vegans to get vitamin D is from fortified foods. Check the nutrition facts panel on the labels of foods fortified with vitamin D, such as breakfast cereals, soy beverages, and some calcium-fortified juices. Your prenatal vitamin should also ensure that you are receiving the amount of vitamin D you need daily for a healthy pregnancy. The requirement for pregnant women is 5 mcg per day.

Iron

Regardless of whether you are a vegetarian, it is likely that you don't get enough iron. This nutrient is often lacking in women's diets. As a result, during pregnancy, women are often prescribed a prenatal vitamin and mineral supplement that includes iron to meet their increased needs and to prevent iron-deficiency anemia. As a pregnant vegetarian, it can be difficult to get enough absorbable iron to meet your daily needs.

Some plant foods do contain iron. Called nonheme iron, it is not absorbed as well as the iron found in animal foods, or heme iron. The challenge for vegetarians is to improve the absorption of nonheme iron foods. You can start by consuming iron-rich plant sources every day, such as legumes, iron-fortified cereals and breads, whole-wheat and whole-grain products, tofu, some dark-green leafy vegetables, seeds, nuts, tempeh, prune juice, blackstrap molasses, and dried fruit.

If your vegetarian diet allows you to consume eggs, keep in mind that they too contain nonheme iron. You can increase your body's absorption of nonheme iron by including a vitamin C–rich food with these nonheme iron sources at every meal, such as orange juice and other citrus juices, citrus fruits, broccoli, tomatoes, and green or red peppers. If you are a semi-vegetarian, eat a little meat, poultry, or fish with nonheme iron sources to help your body better absorb the iron.

Vitamin B$_{12}$

Vitamin B$_{12}$ is mainly found in animal foods. Because plant foods are not a reliable source of vitamin B$_{12}$, it can be a concern for vegetarians, especially vegans. Vitamin B$_{12}$ is important for helping the body make red blood cells and use fats and amino acids. It is also part of the structure of every cell in the body. The body only needs small amounts of vitamin B$_{12}$. Because it is stored and recycled in the body, a deficiency in the short term is not likely. Over time, however, a deficiency of vitamin B$_{12}$ can result in anemia.

ALERT

Some products, such as seaweed, algae, spirulina, tempeh, and miso, are not good sources of vitamin B$_{12}$ even though their packages may make a different claim. The vitamin B$_{12}$ that is contained in these products is inactive and is not in a form that the body can utilize.

Every day, vegans need to consume at least one (preferably more) serving of foods fortified with vitamin B$_{12}$, such as fortified breakfast cereals, soy milk products, rice milk beverages, or meat substitute products such as vegetarian burgers.

If you are a vegetarian who eats dairy and eggs, vitamin B_{12} intake should not be a problem as long as you consume the recommended number of daily food group servings. Vitamin B_{12} is usually a standard vitamin included in most prenatal supplements. Most prenatal vitamin supplements contain cyancobalamin, the form of vitamin B_{12} most easily absorbed by the body.

Zinc

It is tough to get enough zinc when you do not consume meat, poultry, or seafood of any kind. Zinc can be found in eggs and milk, as well as other dairy products. You can also get zinc from plant foods, though it is not absorbed as well as the zinc from animal foods. Zinc-containing plant foods include whole-wheat bread, whole grains, bran, wheat germ, legumes and peas, tofu, seeds, and nuts. Most well-balanced vegetarian diets supply enough zinc, but you should make sure that you consume sufficient amounts. Even mild deficiencies can have an effect on mental performance for both adults and children. Though your prenatal vitamin contains zinc, you should also be sure to get zinc from foods in your diet.

The Power of Protein

When you become pregnant, your protein needs increase by 30 percent. Protein can be found in both animal and plant foods, which makes it easy for both meat-eating and vegetarian women to get all of the protein they need. If you are a vegan, as long as you eat a wide variety of plant foods including whole grains, cereals, legumes, and soy products at each meal, you too should have no problem consuming all of the protein you need for a healthy pregnancy.

Protein is considered a macronutrient because it provides the body with energy, or calories. Protein is part of every cell in the body. Your body requires a constant supply of protein to repair body cells as they wear out. During pregnancy, you need protein to make new cells. Your body's tissues are all unique because of the differing amino acid patterns in their proteins. Amino acids are the building blocks of proteins. Your body uses about twenty different amino acids to make body proteins. Of those, nine are considered essential—your body cannot make them, and you must get them from the foods you eat. The others are considered nonessential amino acids because your body does make them as long as you consume enough essential amino acids and enough calories each day. Animal foods such as meat, poultry, fish, eggs, milk, cheese, and yogurt contain all nine essential amino acids. These foods are said to contain "complete proteins" or "high-quality proteins." Plant foods, on the other hand, contain essential amino acids, but not all nine together. These sources are said to be "incomplete proteins."

FACT

Soy is the exception to the incomplete protein rule. Soy is the only plant food that is a complete protein and contains all nine of the essential amino acids.

Gone are the days when vegans were instructed to eat foods in special combinations at each meal to make sure they were getting the right mix of essential amino acids to make proteins. Instead, vegans need only make sure they are eating a balanced diet that includes a wide variety of plant foods and that provides enough calories each and every day. If you are a vegan, this eating plan will ensure you are receiving all of the essential amino acids in needed amounts each day to make the proteins that your body needs. It is more important to think about your total day's intake rather than each individual meal's.

Omega-3 Essential Fatty Acids

Fats are made up of two types: saturated and unsaturated. Unsaturated fats include monounsaturated and polyunsaturated. Two polyunsaturated fatty acids, linoleic acid (omega-6) and alpha-linolenic acid (omega-3), are considered essential because the body cannot make them. Omega-3 fatty acids are essential fats that can be very heart-healthy as well as vital to the development of a baby's brain and nerves. They are also vital to eye development, growth, and vision. In addition, researchers are studying the question of whether omega-3 fatty acids are helpful in preventing preterm labor and possibly protecting against postpartum depression.

Sources of Omega-3 Fatty Acids

Vegetarians are advised to consume omega-3 fatty acids from eggs as well as from plant-based ingredients such as canola oil, soybean oil, walnuts, walnut oil, ground flaxseed (which you can add to baked goods or smoothies), flaxseed oil, soybeans, wheat germ, and other nuts and seeds. For vegetarians who sometimes consume fish, fatty fish such as salmon, mackerel, herring, trout, tuna, and sardines also supply omega-3 fatty acids.

CHAPTER 7

Weighing In

Comparisons between different pregnancies and the weight gained with each may make for great social conversation, but should never be considered a standard by which to gauge your own healthy weight gain while pregnant. Every pregnancy is as different as every mom, and trying to mimic someone else's ideal pregnancy can be a dangerous path to travel. Your goal for weight gain in pregnancy should focus on the needs of *your* body and *your* baby.

BMI

Your Body Mass Index is commonly referred to as your BMI by health and fitness professionals. Rather than looking at your weight as a number that you feel should be higher or lower, or aiming for an arbitrary weight that you assume is where you should be, your BMI takes into account your height and weight in order to determine whether your weight falls into a category that is healthy or unhealthy. With five categories that range from "underweight" to "severely obese," calculating your BMI can be an easy way to determine whether you have risks for weight-related health issues and need to focus more heavily on reaching a more optimal weight range with less associated risks.

To figure out your BMI, use the following formula:

Weight (pounds) ÷ 2.2 = weight in kilograms (kg)
Height (inches) ÷ 39.37 = height in meters (m)
Weight (kg) ÷ height (m) squared = BMI

Check your BMI against the following chart to see where your present weight places you for risk of health problems related to your body weight:

BMI	Risk for health problems related to body weight
20–25	Very low risk
26–30	Low risk
31–35	Moderate risk
36–39	High risk
40–plus	Very high risk

If your BMI is greater than 30, you should consult your personal physician for further evaluation, especially before becoming pregnant.

Determine Your Caloric Needs

There are many different methods for estimating caloric needs. It is important to remember that these methods result only in estimates; still, you can get a general idea of the number of calories your body needs. Everyone's caloric needs differ, depending on factors such as age, gender, size, body composition, basal metabolic rate, and physical activity.

Basal metabolic rate (BMR) is the number of calories your body would burn if you were at rest all day. By figuring your basal metabolic rate, you know the minimum number of calories you must consume to maintain your weight. On average, a moderately active woman needs between 1,800 and 2,200 calories per day. A pregnant woman needs about 2,500 calories after the first trimester. However, because you don't spend every day lying in bed, you have additional calorie needs on top of your basal rate. The next section describes how to determine the number of calories you should ingest every day.

You Do the Math

Use this simple equation to figure your basic calorie needs:

1. First, figure your basal metabolic rate to get the minimum number of calories your body needs to maintain a healthy weight. To do this, multiply your healthy weight (in pounds) by 10. For instance, a woman whose healthy weight is 165 pounds would have a basal metabolic rate of 1,650—in other words, this woman needs to take in a minimum of 1,650 calories to maintain her body weight.
2. Figure how many additional calories you need to sustain your level of physical activity. To do this, choose the activity level from the following list that best describes you and take the appropriate percentage of your basal metabolic rate.
   - **Sedentary**—You mainly engage in low-intensity activities throughout your day, such as sitting, driving a car, lying down, sleeping, standing, typing, or reading. Take 20 percent of your basal metabolic rate (multiply by 0.2).
   - **Light activity**—Your day includes light exercise, such as walking, but for no more than two hours of your day. Take 30 percent of your basal metabolic rate (multiply by 0.3).
   - **Moderate activity**—You engage in moderate exercise throughout the day, such as heavy housework, gardening, dancing, with very little sitting. Take 40 percent of your basal metabolic rate (multiply by 0.4).

- **High activity**—You engage in active physical sports or have a labor-intensive job, such as construction work, on a daily basis. Take 50 percent of your basal metabolic rate (multiply by 0.5).

3. Figure out how many additional calories you need to sustain your body's digestion and absorption of nutrients. To do this, add your results from steps 1 and 2, then take 10 percent of the total (multiply by 0.1).

4. To find your total calorie needs, add your basal metabolic rate from step 1, the calories to sustain your level of physical activity from step 2, and the number of calories needed for digestion from step 3.

   Take the example of the 165-pound woman from step 1, with the basal metabolic rate of 1,650. She is moderately active, which means she needs an additional 660 calories to sustain her activity level. She needs 231 calories to fuel her body's digestion and food absorption processes $(1,650+ 660×0.1=231)$. Adding those values gives us a total of 2,541, which is the total number of calories a moderately active 165-pound woman should ingest to maintain her weight.

5. To account for the additional calories you need to sustain your body weight during pregnancy, add 300 to the total from step 4. This final value represents your estimated basic calorie needs.

A Little Extra Help

Doing the math will only give you an estimate of your calorie needs. Some women have special needs. If you are having problems figuring out your calorie needs, or if you are not sure what to eat to get those extra calories in, don't hesitate to contact a registered dietitian to help you out. Some women may need a little extra nutritional help to ensure they are getting everything that they need. It is recommended that you seek extra help if you are younger than seventeen or older than thirty-five, pregnant with more than one baby, underweight or overweight prior to becoming pregnant, a strict vegetarian, lactose intolerant, gaining too much or too little during pregnancy, having trouble eating due to nausea and/or vomiting, on a special diet due to allergies, diabetes, or gastrointestinal or digestive disorder, or if you have suffered with eating disorders. Don't go it alone if you are not sure what to do. Nutrition and calorie intake is vital to a healthy baby and a healthy pregnancy. Never hesitate to ask for help!

Healthy Pregnancy Weight Gain

The health and weight of your baby at birth depend greatly on how much weight you gain over the course of your pregnancy. The weight of your baby factors into your weight gain, but your body also gains weight through its increase in blood volume—about 50 percent—as well as muscle, fluid, and tissue. Your body weight increases at a different rate depending on your stage of pregnancy. During the first trimester, weight gain is slow, only about 2 to 4 pounds for the whole time period. During the last six months, weight gain should increase to about ½ to 1 pound per week, depending on your total target weight gain. Even though all women differ slightly, it is best to gain weight at a steady pace.

Trimester	Weight Gain
First trimester (1–3 months)	2 to 4 pounds
Second trimester (4–6 months)	12 to 14 pounds
Third trimester (7–9 months)	8 to 10 pounds

Your body weight before pregnancy will help to determine a healthy weight gain for you during pregnancy. The American College of Obstetricians and Gynecologists recommends the following target weight gains for healthy women. Keep in mind that these are only guidelines and that every woman is unique.

Pre-Pregnancy Weight	Suggested Weight Gain
Normal weight (BMI of 19.8 to 26)	25 to 35 pounds
Overweight (BMI 26 to 29)	15 to 25 pounds
Obese (BMI greater than 29)	At least 15 pounds
Underweight (BMI of less than 19.8)	28 to 40 pounds

Because all women are different, suggested weight gains are expressed in ranges. Shoot for your target weight gain, and if you are not sure where your pre-pregnancy weight falls, speak to your doctor or calculate your pre-pregnancy BMI.

Your goal should be to maintain a steady weight gain throughout your pregnancy. Your baby requires a daily supply of essential nutrients during your entire pregnancy, and that comes from what you eat every day. Expect your weight gain to fluctuate a bit from week to week and to gain more or less depending on the stage of your pregnancy. However, if your weight fluctuates too much or changes suddenly, that could be a warning sign. Be aware of some of the following red flags:

- Gaining more than 3 pounds in any one week during your second trimester
- Gaining more than 2 pounds in any one week during your third trimester
- Not gaining any weight for more than two weeks in a row at any time during the fourth through the eighth months
- Gaining more weight than you anticipated (given that you are diligent about sticking to a well-balanced, healthy meal plan daily)

If you experience any of these or other warning signs, you should discuss it with your doctor at your next visit.

Women who are African-American or in their teenage years (younger than eighteen) are advised to gain toward the upper limit of the weight range to help decrease the risk for delivering a low birth-weight baby. Taller women should shoot for the higher end of the weight gain ranges, and shorter women (62 inches or under) should shoot for the lower end of the range for weight gain.

Don't be obsessive about weighing yourself every day. Your weight can fluctuate too much from day to day to pinpoint possible problems this way. Instead, make regular doctor's visits, and weigh yourself at home every week or two to make sure you are on the right track.

Dieting During Pregnancy

Pregnancy is not the time to worry about losing weight, no matter what your pre-pregnancy weight was. Nor is it the time to worry about spoiling your girlish figure. Once you become pregnant, your focus should be on gaining the recommended amount of weight and on living a healthier lifestyle for a healthy pregnancy. It is the time to eat healthy and stay fit, not skimp on calories. Your baby is constantly growing and needs constant nourishment. You can think about weight loss and reaching a healthier weight once your pregnancy is over and you have finished breastfeeding your baby.

FACT

Never take any type of diet pill or weight-loss supplement, even those claiming to be "safe and natural," while trying to conceive or once you are pregnant. These can be harmful to the fetus.

Even when you are trying to conceive, it is advisable to stay away from extreme fad diets since you may not know you are pregnant immediately. Fad diets can be too low in the calories and essential nutrients you need from the very start of pregnancy. If you need to reach a healthier weight before pregnancy, do it by sticking to a low-fat, high-fiber, well-balanced diet and exercising regularly.

If you've had gastric bypass surgery, doctors recommend that you stay at a stable weight for six months before trying to conceive. Also, be sure to see a nutritionist to determine your specific nutritional needs during pregnancy.

Dieting either before or during pregnancy can lead to nutritional deficiencies that can affect the proper development of your baby. Dieting by decreasing your caloric intake can lead to too little weight gain during pregnancy, which can lead to problems such as premature labor and delivering a low birth-weight baby. Do not try to lose weight in order to keep from gaining too much during your pregnancy. Bigger women are unlikely to gain as much weight during pregnancy as smaller women might. Keep your weight gain to the advised levels, and do not try to lose weight!

Eating Disorders

Maintaining a positive body image can be tough for any woman. During pregnancy, body image concerns seem to become even more prevalent. Eating disorders such as anorexia and bulimia seem to be more prevalent in women and tend to peak around the childbearing years. For women who are already struggling with an eating disorder, pregnancy can be a difficult time that can cause the disorder to worsen. Any type of eating disorder can affect the reproductive process and be dangerous during pregnancy.

Types of Eating Disorders

Anorexia nervosa is an eating disorder in which a person starves herself by eating little to no food. These people have a strong fear of body fat and weight gain. The most dangerous hazard of anorexia is starvation and its extreme health consequences. Obviously, for someone who is pregnant and whose food intake is responsible for supporting a fetus, anorexia could be detrimental. Not eating during pregnancy deprives the baby of essential nutrients she needs for proper growth and development.

Bulimia nervosa is an eating disorder in which a person binges, or consumes a very large amount of food all at once, and then purges by forcing herself to vomit or by taking laxatives or diuretics (water pills). The dangers of bulimia nervosa include electrolyte imbalances from repeated vomiting. Many people with bulimia are able to maintain normal body weight, making the disorder more difficult to detect.

FACT

Eating disorders can affect fertility *and* reduce a woman's chance of becoming pregnant. Most women with anorexia do not have regular menstrual cycles, and about half of all women with bulimia do not have normal cycles. This irregular menstrual cycle can make it extremely challenging to get pregnant.

Binge-eating disorder is very common in women. With a binge-eating disorder, a person is unable to control the desire to overeat. These people are not necessarily overweight or obese. The food they binge on is usually not nutritious but instead filled with fat, sugar, and calories.

Effects on Pregnancy

Eating disorders can have a very negative impact on pregnancy. There are numerous complications that can occur and put you and your baby at higher risk. Some of these complications include the following:

- Premature labor
- Low birth-weight baby
- Stillbirth or fetal death
- Higher risk of C-section
- Low Apgar scores (the Apgar score is an evaluation of a newborn's physical condition after delivery)
- Delayed fetal growth respiratory problems
- Gestational diabetes
- Complications during labor
- Low amniotic fluid, miscarriage
- Preeclampsia (toxemia)
- Birth defects

Pregnancy can exacerbate other medical problems that are related to eating disorders, such as liver, kidney, and cardiac damage. Women who struggle with bulimia usually gain excess weight during pregnancy, putting them at higher risk for hypertension or high blood pressure. Women who struggle with eating disorders through pregnancy also tend to have higher rates of postpartum depression, and they can have difficulty with breastfeeding.

If a women abuses laxatives, diuretics, or other medications to help get rid of calories during pregnancy, she can cause harm to her baby in many ways. These types of over-the-counter medications can also rid the body of valuable fluids and nutrients before they can be used to nourish and feed the baby. Over-the-counter medications, even if they are considered safe during pregnancy, can be dangerous when used in this manner or when used excessively.

How to Cope

If you struggle with an eating disorder, you may be at an increased risk for several complications during your pregnancy. It is vital that you take action immediately to increase your chances of having a healthy pregnancy and a healthy baby. You can still take steps to help ensure a normal pregnancy. If you are able to eat healthily and gain the normal weight that you should throughout your pregnancy, you should have no greater risk of complications or birth defects than anyone else. Your first and most important step is to seek medical and psychological help with your disorder, if you have not already done so.

ESSENTIAL

Even if you feel your eating disorder is a thing of the past, keep in mind that physical and emotional changes during pregnancy can trigger depression and a relapse of an eating disorder. Don't take it lightly. If you had an eating disorder in the past, talk to your doctor and consider visiting a therapist prior to and during your pregnancy.

Follow some of these guidelines if you struggle with an eating disorder and want to become pregnant or have discovered that you are pregnant.

Before pregnancy, do the following:

- If you have an eating disorder and have not yet searched for professional help, that needs to be your first step—before you even begin to consider pregnancy.
- Achieve and maintain a normal and healthy weight.
- Consult with your doctor and receive a medical checkup. Ask about prenatal vitamins.
- Meet with a dietitian, and start a healthy pregnancy diet. Once you become pregnant, the baby will take from your own nutritional stores. If they are not built up, it could cause problems for both you and your baby.
- Continue any counseling, both individual and group, that you are involved with.

- If you have already gone through counseling, it would be a good idea to go back to your therapist to discuss concerns about body image that may surface during pregnancy.
- Seriously consider and discuss with your therapist the implications and complications of becoming pregnant before you have successfully recovered.

During pregnancy, do the following:

- Have a prenatal visit early in your pregnancy and discuss with your doctor your past and/or present struggles with eating disorders. The more honest you are with your doctor, the more he can help.
- Shoot to achieve an essential and healthy weight gain. The closer you are to a normal weight gain, the better your chance of having a healthy baby.
- Continue to visit with a dietitian to receive instruction on eating a healthy diet, how many calories are necessary, and making the right choices. Seek out a dietitian with experience in eating disorders.
- Do whatever you can to normalize your eating and eliminate purging activities.
- Continue to seek counseling to address your eating disorder and any underlying concerns. A therapist can help you through the difficult times of your pregnancy when your body begins to change.

Just as important as before and during pregnancy is the care you continue to receive after your baby is born. Women with eating disorders are more susceptible to postpartum depression, so continue with your counseling. Eating disorder behaviors can also hinder your breastfeeding efforts, so don't allow yourself to fall back into unhealthy pre-pregnancy habits. To find out more information on eating disorders, visit the National Eating Disorders Association website at *www.nationaleatingdisorders.org*, or the Renfrew Center at *www.renfrew.org*.

CHAPTER 8

Essential Exercise

Keeping yourself healthy and fit prior to pregnancy is important, but while pregnant, exercise is essential! From beginning to end, and even following your pregnancy, the exercise you do while pregnant has lasting effects on your health, the health of your pregnancy, and the development of your baby. The benefits are enough to get any mom moving, even if you feel like exercise isn't your "thing"!

The Physiological Effects

The physiological benefits of exercise on pregnancy are great. Not only can exercise improve the course of your pregnancy and of your labor, but it can also help you reduce stress. The benefits also go well into the postpartum period and beyond.

FACT

Backache in pregnancy is one of the most common complaints women have. Not only does exercise help with alleviating back pain, but it also helps prevent back pain from occurring to begin with. Exercise also makes caring for your baby easier after the birth because your muscles are more used to being held appropriately.

Body awareness is a key component to exercise in pregnancy (and pregnancy in general!). As you begin to exercise, your body awareness increases. This attention to your body can help you become more attuned to problems before they become larger issues. This can in turn lead to an increase in attention to proper body mechanics and body posture, both of which are key to a comfortable pregnancy.

The Physical Benefits of Exercise

The improved body awareness that you gain from exercising will help you manage the physical symptoms of pregnancy with greater ease. This directly corresponds with feeling more comfortable as your body goes through the many changes of the three trimesters. Exercising will also decrease the number of physical complaints commonly associated with pregnancy.

Other physical benefits of exercise in pregnancy include:

- Decrease in headaches
- Decrease in shortness of breath
- Improved digestion
- Improved bowel function
- Increased sense of well-being

- Decreased tendency toward depression
- Maintained or improved cardiovascular strength
- Increased pelvic floor strength
- Improved posture
- Better sense of control over body issues

ESSENTIAL

The physical complaints of pregnancy are many. Among the most often-heard complaints are fatigue, backache, digestion problems, constipation, and swelling. Exercise can help you prevent many of these complaints for a variety of reasons.

Reducing Fatigue and Strength Building

The physical movements of exercise can help you combat the fatigue that is so common in the first and third trimesters. Additionally, exercise helps alleviate problems with insomnia that can plague pregnant women at all stages of pregnancy and recovery.

When you physically utilize your body during the day, your body responds by requiring a recuperation period. The physical demands of exercise, even when not intense, will also help you clear your mind and rest more easily at night.

Certain exercises also increase the strength and the flexibility of your body, which will be very handy advantages for the physical demands of pregnancy and labor. This added strength and mobility will also make the tasks of caring for a newborn seem less extreme.

Blood Volume Increase

When you are pregnant, you experience an increase in your blood volume—as much as 50 percent of your blood volume with one baby and more if you are carrying multiples. Exercise also helps increase the circulation of your blood, which can prevent a number of circulatory issues common to pregnancy: varicose veins of the legs and rectum (hemorrhoids), blood clots that occur during pregnancy and after, and some forms of swelling associated with pregnancy.

The Psychological Effects

By now, you have read a lot of information about the physical benefits of exercise for you and your baby in different periods during the child-bearing years. But there are many emotional and mental benefits as well to gain from exercise. It has long been shown that, in general, exercising helps to lower your stress levels. This stress reduction is very important during such a tense, albeit happy, time in your life.

There is an increased pride in your pregnancy and your pregnant body when you are physically meeting your body's needs through exercise. This sense of confidence and self-esteem that comes from exercise helps you envision your newly rounding figure with pride and pleasure. No longer do you see yourself as a "beached whale" awaiting the delivery of your calf. You now see the beauty and function of your new pregnant form. This is just another benefit of knowing the body you live in.

Finally, as exercise becomes a part of your way of life, it becomes a habit—a healthy habit that can be shared as a family. Exercising moms rarely just quit exercising after the birth of their babies. They begin exercising *with* their babies. This starts the baby on a lifelong journey to seek out fitness for himself or herself, because it is what he or she has learned by Mom's great example.

Labor and Birth Benefits

While people tend to want immediate gratification from everything they do, exercise in pregnancy doesn't always fall into this category. Sometimes it can be difficult to get up and exercise when the benefits aren't seen immediately. However, the exercises you do in pregnancy will certainly affect how you give birth when the time comes.

Having a well-toned and fit body for labor has its advantages. If you have been used to the physical rigors of exercise, you will tend to do better in labor. You will be more prepared for the physical demands placed on your body. The muscles that have been prepared with the strength that you will need for pushing, and perhaps even specifically for the task of labor and birth, are not only stronger as a result of exercise but are also more easily put into action when they are exercised on a regular basis.

Beyond the feelings of having more strength and stamina, there are some specific benefits to you for exercising in pregnancy. Studies have shown that women who exercise during pregnancy often have shorter labors. These women also tend to require cesarean surgery less often, as well as experiencing a decrease in the use of forceps and vacuum extractors. By decreasing the risks of surgery and instrumental deliveries, you will also speed your recovery period.

ESSENTIAL

Some childbirth classes will offer a few prenatal exercises to incorporate into your regular exercise routine. These exercises are usually specially designed to prepare specific muscles in your body for labor and birth. An example might be teaching the class about squatting. It's a great exercise to strengthen your legs and glutes, but is also the perfect position to give birth in as it opens the pelvic outlet by an additional 10 percent.

Postpartum Advantages

Possibly some of the most surprising benefits of exercise in pregnancy are the postpartum benefits. If you've spent time building strength and flexibility during pregnancy, you will tend to have an easier recovery period after the birth of your baby. Coupled with the fact that you will tend to have an easier birth with fewer cesareans and episiotomies, it makes sense.

Not only is exercise beneficial in terms of your weight loss but in your body tone and fitness levels in general. Returning to your pre-pregnancy body is a huge issue for women in the postpartum period. When you stay fit before birth, you have a huge leap ahead of the crowd toward getting your old body back. There also seems to be a protective benefit from postpartum depression when you have exercised during pregnancy.

Benefits for Baby

In the past, one of the main concerns about exercise during pregnancy was that it would have a negative effect on your baby. Some researchers predicted growth restriction, oxygen reduction, and other scary outcomes for babies born to moms who exercised. To the contrary, researchers have now found that there are many physical and psychological benefits for a baby when Mom exercises during pregnancy.

As you become more aware of your pregnant body and your baby, you focus on taking proper care of that body and baby. By watching how and what you eat, you decrease the risks of preterm labor. The decrease in preterm birth rates alone prevents many neonatal deaths, as preterm birth is one of the leading causes of death in newborns.

QUESTION

How can I monitor my baby's well-being while I'm pregnant?
Your practitioner will monitor your baby in a couple of ways during your pregnancy. One way will be by measuring the heart rate; another is the growth rate as judged by the growth of your uterus. Your baby's normal heart rate will probably be between 120 and 160 beats per minute (bpm). After twenty weeks, your uterus will generally measure the same number in centimeters as the number of weeks you are pregnant, within a week or two; for example, if you are twenty-two weeks pregnant, your measurement would be expected to be between 20 and 24 cm. The measurements taken are in centimeters, from the pubic bone to the top of the uterus.

Healthier Placenta

The improved blood circulation of the mother through exercise can help grow a healthier placenta, which is the baby's lifeline during pregnancy, as it uses the placenta to get nutrients and oxygen and to expel waste products. The heartier the placenta, the healthier the baby will be.

Improved Labor Tolerance

Babies of mothers who exercise also seem to tolerate labor better. These babies are used to having Mom work hard while exercising, so that when it is time for Mom to have contractions, it is just another workout for them. This tolerance level has also been shown to decrease the incidence of meconium (baby's first stool) in the amniotic fluid at birth. Having too much meconium in the amniotic fluid is potentially life-threatening and something you would prefer to avoid.

Leaner, Healthier Babies

If you exercise during pregnancy, your baby will tend to be of a lower birth weight. While this might seem like a negative outcome, the lower weight is not from fetal growth restriction, but rather the reduction in deposits of unnecessary fat for the baby. These leaner babies at birth are also healthier and leaner later in life. Some studies even report that babies born to mothers who exercised during pregnancy were easier to care for after birth and seemed to adjust to their environments more readily.

Perhaps these babies are reported to be easier because the rocking motions associated with maternal exercise during pregnancy offered stimulation to enhance baby's brain development. One study, "Morphometric and neurodevelopmental outcome at age five years of the offspring of women who continued to exercise regularly throughout pregnancy" (*J. Pediatr.* 1996 Dec; 129[6]:856–63), shows that these babies actually had better language and intelligence scores at five years of life.

Why Exercise Is Different During Pregnancy

As with many other aspects of your lifestyle that change with pregnancy, your new body and new responsibilities make exercise very different from when you're not expecting. Simply knowing what physical changes can possibly lead to potentially dangerous situations can help you understand how to avoid them and keep yourself and your baby safe from harm.

Center of Gravity

Your center of gravity is located in the middle of your abdomen, just above your belly button or umbilicus. Usually, you will not notice any changes to this area until you are into your third or fourth month of pregnancy. Once your uterus has begun to grow out of your pelvic region, your center of gravity will shift upward.

This shift itself is not painful, nor is it cause for alarm. In fact, you will probably not even notice the changes taking place, as it is a gradual process. Your body will naturally adapt to most center of gravity changes. What you do need to watch for is the natural loss of balance that may occur that will probably continue throughout pregnancy, steadily growing as your abdomen does.

ALERT

It's always wise to wear the appropriate footwear. This goes for times of exercise as well as in everyday life. A simple fall can stress you, leave you feeling unsteady, or (at worst) seriously harm you or your baby.

Many women report that they feel off balance as their abdomen grows. You might experience this as well. The biggest danger is that the shift makes falls more likely. The good news is that even a serious fall is generally not harmful to your baby. He or she is tucked safely away in the amniotic sac, blissfully unaware of your most recent belly flop. A shift in the center of gravity is more likely to cause problems with your posture as well. Posture is key to feeling good and looking good during your pregnancy. While exercising, simply be aware of your abdomen and try to remain conscious of the movements you are making and how you are moving. This awareness can help with any problems you might experience.

Joints and Flexibility

As with everything in pregnancy, your joints are also affected. This includes your elbows, shoulders, hips, knees, wrists, and ankles. The usual culprits, your hormones, namely relaxin, are to blame for the increased risk of injury to these areas.

Joints can be injured very easily during pregnancy. Using warmup sessions and cool-downs, you can greatly reduce the risk of harming the joints during pregnancy. These exercises also have the added benefits of working your range of motion.

Trust Your Body

We have all heard the "no pain, no gain" mantra that is so common in health centers today. And as a society, we all seem too eager to buy into that theory. While it is true that you have to expend energy to get the benefit of exercise, pain has no place in exercise, particularly during pregnancy.

Pain

Pain is your body's way of saying something is wrong. When you are pregnant, it is even more important that you pay attention to these signals from your body. Remember, your baby is counting on you to listen.

Pain should be something that makes you stop exercising immediately. No matter where the location of the pain or what the feeling is like, stop doing whatever you are doing. Sometimes pain is a signal that you have a hurt muscle or a leg cramp. While these may not have a direct negative effect on your pregnancy, they can harm your body.

This type of cramping pain may be more likely to occur during pregnancy. For example, if you have a leg cramp, it may be a sign that your electrolytes are out of balance and that you need to watch your nutritional intake more closely or stretch more often. An injured muscle could result from your body's release of the hormone relaxin, which helps to facilitate the birth but also has the effect of making injuries more likely.

Falls

Due to the changes in your center of gravity and the hormones coursing through your body, falls may be more likely when pregnant. For this reason, some exercises (e.g., horseback riding) are never recommended during pregnancy.

While you may be at an increased risk for falls, learning to take certain precautions can certainly help reduce this likelihood. During your normal daily life avoid high heels, walk on pathways whenever you can, and avoid uneven surfaces or stones. Whenever you work out, remember to wear the appropriate footwear.

If you do fall, try not to panic. Check yourself out completely before standing back up. In general, your baby is well protected by the amniotic sac in your uterus. However, if you experience any abdominal pain, bleeding, contractions, or changes in the baby's movements, report this immediately to your practitioner.

ESSENTIAL

Remember to eat something a few hours before you work out. The meal you have prior to a workout should be snack-sized with lots of quality nutrition like complex carbs and protein. Some yogurt and a piece of fruit is one example. This will help your body sustain your energy through your fitness session.

Feeling Weak or Dizzy

Feeling weak or dizzy is a sign that you probably need to skip your exercise today. These feelings can be a normal part of your pregnancy, or they may indicate a problem. Sometimes you feel weak from the exhaustion of pregnancy, more typically in the first and third trimesters. Other issues for feeling weak or dizzy would be a dramatic fluctuation in your blood sugar levels.

If you begin to feel weak or lightheaded during your workout, stop immediately. Sit down or lie down. Have someone bring you water. You should not try to drive or walk. If you actually pass out, be sure to call your doctor or midwife as soon as you awake. Call your doctor or midwife right away if the symptoms don't go away within a few minutes. Otherwise, report your symptoms to your practitioner during normal office hours. They may suggest you alter your exercise plan going forward.

Sometimes simply not feeling right is a perfect indicator to stop. It could be you're having an off day. Maybe you've not eaten recently enough or perhaps you're tired. Whatever the reason, listen to your body's signals and stop exercising.

The Talk Test

The "talk test" is one of the simpler ways for you to determine whether or not you are exercising at the right intensity for your body and your baby. It is much easier to do than taking your pulse and can be done without any equipment and at any location.

The only thing you have to do is to ask yourself whether you can carry on a conversation with the person next to you without sounding out of breath or winded. It's as simple as that.

So if, for example, you are out walking with your family or friends in your neighborhood and you are discussing weekend plans, can you do this without huffing and puffing? Or do you sound like you are in need of a breathing machine? If you can carry on the conversation without being winded, you are exercising at the appropriate intensity for you.

ALERT

While exercising, it is normal to be somewhat out of breath. You should exert yourself enough to work your heart and lungs during your exercise sessions, but not to a dangerous extent. The difference between a good windedness and being too short of breath is going to be your ability to carry on a conversation, either real or imagined. Talk to yourself if you need to, just to be sure you're not pushing yourself too hard.

Now, what do you do if you are winded? Very simple—slow it down. This doesn't mean coming to a complete stop (unless it's severe), but rather shorten your strides when walking and drop the pace, even if this means you fall behind the group. If you are doing aerobics, you might consider doing only leg motions and keeping your arms at your sides instead of including them in the workout, too. If that doesn't work, you can also try walking in place until you can talk at a normal conversational pattern.

When conversation has returned to a normal pace, slowly add speed or activity to what you are doing, being careful not to overexert yourself again. Remember, as you exercise more, your tolerance will increase. The walking pace that winded you last week might be perfect this week.

When Not to Exercise

While there are not many reasons that exercise would be contraindicated during pregnancy, it is important to know what to look for in terms of protecting yourself. In general, here are some problems that you may experience that would signal you to stop exercise during portions or all of your pregnancy.

Bleeding

About 30 to 40 percent of women will experience some form of bleeding during pregnancy. The majority of these women, more than 60 percent, will go on to carry a healthy baby to the end of pregnancy. However, it is wise to find out the source of the bleeding, which will determine whether or not you can exercise.

FACT

Placenta previa, detected via ultrasound prior to twenty weeks of gestation, may or may not interfere with the birth process. As you enter the second trimester, the body of the uterus begins a major growth spurt, often helping the placenta move from the cervical region in 95 percent of women. If the placenta does not move far enough away by the end of your pregnancy, your baby will be born via a cesarean surgery to ensure the safety of both mom and baby.

For example, the cervix region becomes much more vascular during pregnancy. Sometimes something as simple as a vaginal exam or sexual intercourse can cause the cervix to bleed slightly. While this is definitely scary, it does not necessarily mean an impending miscarriage or other problems with the pregnancy. However, bleeding from the uterus, or between the uterus and the placenta, also called a *partial abruption*, would be a reason not to exercise during this pregnancy until the issues were resolved and your doctor or midwife gave you the go-ahead.

Placenta previa is a condition in which part of or the entire placenta covers the opening of the uterus, the cervix. This can lead to bleeding, with or without pain, as well as pregnancy loss and other trauma to the pregnancy. There may not be an opportunity for you to exercise during this type of pregnancy because of the inherent risks. Ask your provider about how this will affect your pregnancy and birth. You might also ask how often and how they intend to monitor the location of the placenta. Many times this condition will spontaneously resolve itself during the second trimester as the body of the uterus grows, helping to move the placenta away from the cervix.

History of Preterm Labor

If you have previously given birth to a baby before thirty-seven weeks, you will want to talk to your practitioner about exercise. In certain cases, your previous birth may have had a non-repeating factor that caused you to have your baby early. This means that this particular pregnancy is not at a higher risk for preterm birth. Some practitioners, however, will advise that exercise for the first portion of pregnancy is best avoided to confirm the fact that it was a non-repeating factor. And then again, they may advise taking it easy during the later portion of pregnancy.

Contractions

The rhythmic tightening of the uterus that leads to cervical changes is not good; if you feel it, you should discontinue exercising immediately. These contractions are an indicator of preterm labor, even if they are not painful or even noticeable. Any regularly occurring contractions you feel prior to thirty-seven weeks of pregnancy should be immediately reported to your doctor or midwife.

ESSENTIAL

Timing contractions is very simple. Using a watch with a second hand, make a note of when a contraction begins. When the contraction ends, make note of that time as well. The third number to write down will be when the next contraction starts. The period from the beginning of the first contraction to the beginning of the second contraction is how far apart your contractions are. How long they last is from the beginning of one contraction until it ends.

It can be perfectly normal to have slight contractions for about twenty to thirty minutes after exercising. However, the contractions that do not stop after this short period of time or those that become very painful or intense need to be reported to your practitioner. Drinking water and lying on your left side should also help contractions decrease in frequency.

Incompetent Cervix

Incompetent cervix is a condition in which your cervix dilates prior to being full term. This can happen with or without noticeable contractions. You may have been previously diagnosed with an incompetent cervix in this or a previous pregnancy, in which case you will probably be treated with a cervical cerclage, a stitch placed in the cervix to attempt to delay labor. Exercise is usually contraindicated because of the risk of preterm labor.

Membrane Ruptures

If your water breaks, you will likely be confined to bed rest for the remainder of your pregnancy in an attempt to prevent the preterm birth of your baby. While on bed rest, there may be opportunities to do certain types of physical therapy to help prevent muscle loss. Talk to your medical team about utilizing these services. Regular exercise is simply not possible.

Pregnancy-Induced Hypertension (PIH)

When your blood pressure is elevated in pregnancy, one must worry about the effects on mom and baby. Overall, exercise will tend to lower blood pressure, but during the actual exercise it does raise your blood pressure. Some practitioners advise that you avoid all exercise if you experience any episode of high blood pressure. Other practitioners take a wait-and-see approach, often depending on the severity of your symptoms and the timing of the onset of the symptoms.

Multiple Gestation

When you are carrying more than one baby, it is simply not well studied as to whether or not exercise is acceptable or beneficial. The general consensus is that with twins, moderate exercise in the beginning of pregnancy is acceptable. Since you will be more closely monitored during the second half of pregnancy, you can look for signs of impending preterm birth, like a shortening cervix. This will alert you and your provider to what changes you need to make in your physical activity levels.

In the later portion of pregnancy, exercise will have to be considered on a case-by-case basis. For those women carrying more than two babies, higher order multiples (HOM), greater restrictions on exercise during pregnancy will exist. However, physical therapy and some forms of stretching may be perfectly acceptable. Again, working with your practitioner is the best option.

Some of these conditions might not make exercise impossible for you, though you may wish to consider modifying your program. It's very important to discuss your current fitness status with your doctor or midwife.

CHAPTER 9

Setting Yourself Up for Exercise Success

Before you start, or continue, your prenatal exercise routine, there are a couple of things you can do to make the transition a little easier. From identifying your current fitness level and your goals, to how to fit exercise into your busy schedule and what to wear, you can set yourself up for exercise success by thinking ahead and creating a plan.

Talk to Your Doctor

Talking with your doctor or midwife about exercise might seem way down on your list of things to discuss in the precious few minutes you have during a regular prenatal appointment. But you can't afford *not* to talk about this issue. Looking at the benefits of pregnancy exercise, you now know it is important to exercise, but it is also crucial that you receive guidance from those taking care of you during your pregnancy.

Ask your practitioner his opinion on exercise during pregnancy. Does he seem to agree with the current guidelines for pregnancy fitness released by the American College of Obstetricians and Gynecologists (ACOG)? If he doesn't, ask if there is a specific reason you should not exercise or should not exercise to the extent that you believe you should be able to during this pregnancy.

If he doesn't seem to have an answer that is satisfactory, ask him if he is aware of the latest guidelines from ACOG. If he is not aware, offer to share your copy. This education process can benefit not only you but also other patients who are seeing this practitioner.

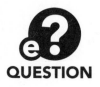

QUESTION

What if my practitioner refuses to follow the new guidelines?
If you and your practitioner can't see eye to eye about exercise, you may have bigger troubles looming. Remember that you are the consumer and that you can switch to a practitioner who is supportive of your decisions concerning exercise. If you can't decide together on this issue, you may not be able to agree on other important decisions later, such as medication during labor, genetic testing, and so on.

Maybe you're one of the lucky women who has a practitioner who is very up to date on the latest exercise guidelines and is actually encouraging you. Perhaps your provider has a belief in exercise that exceeds the ACOG guidelines. Finding a happy medium—the middle of the road that both you and your practitioner can live with—goes both ways. Talking to your doctor or midwife will help you tailor a fitness program for you and your baby that is safe and effective. This will help ensure a healthy and safe pregnancy fitness course.

What's Your Fitness Level?

A fitness level is simply defined as what "shape" your body is in, meaning how fit you are on a cardiovascular level as well as your level of muscle tone. To gauge your fitness level, you might look at how often you exercise. Do you walk every day? Perhaps you take one aerobics class per week. Maybe you get in six exercise sessions a week and if you don't, you feel awful. Each of these categories would represent a different fitness level.

The importance of a fitness evaluation cannot be understated. Choosing a place to start your activity will depend largely on this evaluation. How successful and safe your performance is will also be attributed to the proper determination of your pre-pregnancy fitness level.

QUESTION

What if I've never worked out before?
Don't worry! There will be something for you to do as well. Many women start thinking about exercise as they start their families. You just need to be extra alert and careful about the exercises you choose and watch your body's reactions to those choices.

How Fit Are You?

Finding your fitness level is the first step in any pregnancy or pre-pregnancy exercise program. By using some simple questions about your fitness level, you can then decide on the appropriate place to begin for your current pregnancy. An evaluation should be done with each pregnancy, as your fitness level will change throughout your life.

One of the most important elements of the evaluation, however, will not be which category you are in, but rather your determination and dedication to the exercise program. Remember that intermittent exercise can be more harmful to your body than no exercise at all.

When you exercise irregularly, you're always in the initial phases of exercise. You never really build up to anything, as you can't get past the initial stages of the training. There are also mental reasons why irregular exercise is harmful—because it never gets "any better." You are always doing something that feels difficult to do. This can make you lack the desire to exercise and can also make you more prone to injury.

Let's look at three main fitness levels—sedentary, moderately active, and athletic—and determine where you fit in:

Sedentary

If you are sedentary, you probably have not been participating in any type of formal exercise program. You may not exercise at all, or very little. Just because you fit into these criteria does not mean that you are necessarily overweight or unhealthy. You might simply just not be as fit as you potentially could be.

ESSENTIAL

It used to be said that athletes should quit competing when a pregnancy was confirmed. Now we see many pregnant athletes enjoying their sports well into their pregnancy. If you had been athletic prior to becoming pregnant, barring health issues with the pregnancy, there are few reasons you would need to change your athletic ways.

Moderately Active

Do you consider yourself moderately active? If so, you probably enjoy exercise but do not go out of your way to make it a regular part of your life. You may exercise when it is convenient or fits into your social schedule, like a walk in the neighborhood with a friend, or a random aerobics or yoga class. You are more likely to add small portions of exercise to your life, like walking short distances rather than driving, or parking in the back of the parking lot. This category is more for the social exerciser.

Athletic

Do you value your exercise highly and would you be very lost without your regular routine? Perhaps you go to a regular exercise class or schedule exercise on a near daily basis. You may be a competitive athlete, or perhaps you may compete in more than one sport. This category is not restricted to only professional athletes; many varied people enjoy rigorous exercise.

Assess Yourself

Looking at these three categories of fitness, you might think you fit neatly into one of them. However, you should only use the fitness level category as a starting point. Consulting with a trainer who specializes in pregnant populations or asking your physician, you can get an objective assessment of your fitness that can give you a good idea of where and how you could improve your fitness level. On your own, you can use some simple self-check evaluations to determine your fitness level right in the privacy of your own home.

Professional Evaluation

Some women prefer to have a professional evaluation of their fitness level. This can be done in most major fitness centers, including some hospital gyms. If you are having trouble finding someone to perform this assessment, you might try a professional association that trains fitness instructors or personal trainers. Fitness evaluation is a basic skill of personal trainers and fitness instructors.

FACT

If you choose to have a professional evaluation, be sure to ask your evaluator about her certification in the area of pre- and postnatal fitness and nutrition. Choosing a certified fitness instructor or personal trainer will make a huge difference in your evaluation. Having an evaluator with previous experience working with pregnant women will also make it easier for you to ask questions and trust her advice.

A few practitioners might require a professional evaluation before giving you the go-ahead to exercise. If your doctor or midwife requests one from you, ask if he has a recommendation for where to have your fitness levels tested. In most cases, you will be able to use self-evaluation to figure out where to begin your exercise routine.

Self-Evaluation

Begin your self-evaluation by asking yourself the following questions about your body, your pregnancy, and exercise:

- What injuries have you experienced in the past (including broken bones, accidents, falls, previous surgeries, or other problems)?
- Do you have old injuries that still require nurturing? If so, can you find ways to alter different exercises to accommodate this injury?
- What medical conditions, if any, did you have before your pregnancy (e.g., chronic conditions including high blood pressure, heart disease, diabetes, arthritis, etc.)? Are they under control now? Do you have any specific concerns about these conditions?
- Are you suffering from current pregnancy discomforts (e.g., swelling, nausea, backache, etc.)?
- Have you developed potential complications during pregnancy, like gestational diabetes, anemia, or pregnancy-induced hypertension (PIH)? If so, how can you still fit in exercise? Will there be restrictions on which exercises you are able to complete?

Where to Get Your Groove On

The type of exercise you do will determine, at least in part, where you will exercise. For example, walking can be done outside in the neighborhood, on a treadmill in your house, outside at a track, or even inside at the mall.

Planning your workout venue is smart, but it is always wise to have alternative plans in place should something come up, either weather- or life-related, that would make your location plans change. For example, in the heat of summer many avid outdoor walkers become mall walkers. It is free and air-conditioned!

Fitness Centers

Local gyms can be great for pregnancy fitness routines. A place that's open early morning and late at night, isn't affected by weather conditions, provides child care, and has on-site safety provisions, your local fitness center may be the perfect place for you. Usually providing small rooms for private workouts, group fitness classes that cater to pregnant women, and certified trainers who can assist with any questions you may have, gyms are making a strong effort to provide a comfortable atmosphere for a huge population of potential members who are growing increasingly interested in fitness each and every year. If you know of a local fitness center or have heard other moms speaking highly of one in particular, check it out to see if it fits your wants and needs. If you're not sure of a gym in your area, you can always use the Internet to your advantage to find one close to home and check out reviews of members, too.

Exercising at Home

If you are a person who prefers to work out in your home, there are accommodations to be made there, too. This area of your home should be a place that you can easily change into your workout area, or even better, leave as your workout area. You want a well-ventilated and open space in which to do your workouts.

Which room works best, you ask? If you occasionally do a pregnancy workout video, you will want your space to be near a television and a DVD player. If you like to see the outdoors while doing yoga, choose a spot near a window. The actual room itself is not the question, except when dealing with issues of space and practicality. Nearly any room will do.

ESSENTIAL

Phones, doorbells, and computers—they all have a way of distracting you just when you find the time to work out. Remember that this time is your time for yourself, and do whatever you think is necessary to avoid all unnecessary interruptions for the workout period. This will help ensure a better workout and give you a much-needed break from the hustle and bustle of life.

The flooring surface might be an issue, depending on what type of exercise you choose. You might not have a choice of flooring, but you definitely want to ensure that you remove rugs that you could easily fall on or trip over, as well as pieces of furniture that are too close to the exercise area. (This does not mean moving large pieces of furniture on your own as a part of a weightlifting routine.) Know what accessories, if any, will be needed for your workout and keep them nearby.

Once you have chosen your space, remember to gather supplies before you start. There is nothing more frustrating than having to pause a DVD to run to get a chair for balance, or remembering halfway through your yoga workout that you left your props in the trunk of the car. Also remember to bring your water bottle with you. You might want a towel if you perspire— anything you might need during the course of the workout.

Fitting It In

You know that exercising will be good for you, but between work, carpool, family, to-dos, and the new tired or nauseous challenges of pregnancy, you may find yourself wondering where you could find the time. You're not alone. Not having time to exercise is reported as one of the most common reasons for people to quit exercising. Don't let it be yours. If you find yourself searching for excuses not to exercise, try to remember all of those health benefits to you and your baby that result from regular prenatal exercise . . . and the negative outcomes of not exercising consistently or at all. By implementing just a few quick and easy strategies, you can work exercise into even your busiest of days, and feel great for helping yourself and your baby by doing so.

ESSENTIAL

Picking a gym can be a big decision. You should shop around for a gym that will fit your needs during pregnancy as well as after. For example, don't pick a gym based solely on the prenatal classes. What about a nursery? Can you bring the baby back with you once he or she is born? Look at location in relation to your home or work. What would keep you from coming to the gym? What would make you go?

Making a Schedule

One of the best secrets to finding the time to exercise is to schedule the time. Many women find that if they select a morning time, the exercise gets done. If you wait to do your exercise after work or before bed, things might come up during the day making it easily forgotten. Write the time in your planning calendar—and be faithful to it!

What if you don't quite feel up to it one day? Or what if you have trouble getting out of bed? Simply get up and do a modified program. Perhaps instead of doing an aerobics video, you choose to walk the dog leisurely around the block. You are still committing yourself to exercise.

Scheduling the time to exercise into your day is the best way to ensure that you stick to your plan. Just as you make the time to nourish your body with food, be sure to find time to nourish your body with exercise.

Adding Exercise to Your Daily Life

Perhaps there are times when you simply cannot fit exercise into a hectic life, despite scheduling. As long as this does not become a habit, never fear! Find sneaky ways to add exercise into your schedule, "a little bit here, and a little bit there." You'll probably be surprised at how easy it can be to reach your daily goals with a little creativity and dedication.

- Skip the elevator! You should consider taking the stairs when you can. Even if you can't walk up all sixty flights, walking five of them and then taking the elevator the rest of the way up still gives you quite a workout.
- Walk instead of ride. Rather than spending ten minutes circling the parking lot to find the absolutely best space available, try parking at the back of the parking lot and walking to the store. Not only will this give you exercise, but it often saves you time.
- Take your dog for a much-needed walk. Getting out and enjoying the fresh air can be good for you and Fido, not to mention the added benefits to your body.
- Go the extra step. Are you the type of person who carries things to the stairs or one particular room, and leaves a pile to carry up later? Consider taking your belongings up the stairs or to their rightful spot every time you would normally just pile them up. Six or seven trips up the stairs or to the other end of the house throughout the day is a great way to add to your workout without stressing your time limits or lifestyle. The fringe benefit is that you do not have anything to trip over at the bottom of the stairs and your house could look so clean. Just make

sure you are not carrying heavy loads, following the guidelines of your particular caregiver.

- Work out with housework. Doing dishes, folding laundry, sweeping, mopping, and vacuuming can all be transformed from boring chores to exhilarating workouts. You can do calf raises while washing dishes, squats and lunges while doing laundry, or challenge yourself to a certain number of bicep curls or crunches every time you finish sweeping or mopping a room. If you get creative, you can think of tons of new and exciting ways to create workout opportunities from everyday activities you'd have to do anyway.
- Walk it out! If you work at a desk or in an office, you might try taking a walk during a break period or lunch. Not only will it help you fit exercise in, but it will also get you out of the office and give you a chance to clear your head. Be sure to bring a change of shoes so that you are comfortable and safe when you walk.

Workout Clothes

What you wear while exercising is just as important as watching your form. The right clothing can help protect you from falls, balance problems, overheating, and dehydration. Let's not forget to mention that the right outfit can simply make you more comfortable during your workout.

FACT

Picking the right bra is very important in pregnancy. As your breast development changes, your bra needs will be quite different. Many women experience breast changes early in the first trimester that continue throughout a pregnancy. Bra purchases are important and should not be skimped on. Find a supportive bra that prevents bouncing movements and remember that you may go through one or more bra size changes as your pregnancy progresses.

There is not one *right* type of outfit to wear, but rather the right choice is something that keeps you comfortable, safe, and willing to exercise. When you are not pregnant and you are working out, you may have a favorite type of outfit. You might be a sweat suit type of person, or perhaps you prefer running shorts and a jogging bra. Either way, you can carry this over to your pregnancy workout attire with just a few simple adjustments.

Maternity Fashion

Luckily enough, major retailers and designers have developed full lines of maternity clothing designed specifically for exercise. Pregnancy workout attire is not only readily available and inexpensive, but attractive and feminine, too. Gone are the days that you would have to use your husband's clothes for a home workout, or choose from a slim variety of appealing options. Whatever your taste, you can find maternity clothes for exercise sessions that can make your workouts comfortable, enjoyable, and stylish, too!

Wearing the Proper Clothing

When dressing to work out, remember to dress as you normally would, keeping in mind considerations for your pregnant body. With the increased blood volume circulating in your body, you might become hot more quickly. You will probably want to wear two layers of clothing consisting of a cover shirt that can be easily removed if you become too hot, and a breathe-easy sports bra or well-ventilated top underneath for maximum comfort and ventilation. Two layers are also helpful during your workout, as they will allow you to remove some clothes without having to put a complete halt to your workout session.

Choose clothes that breathe. For example, cotton is great for working out and is particularly valuable in the choice of your underwear or pants. Synthetic materials in this sensitive area can make you more likely to develop a rash or even a yeast infection.

While you don't want your clothes so loose that they end up falling to the floor or showing off a little more skin than you would hope, you'll want to pay attention to the fit of your fitness clothes when you purchase them to ensure they're not too constricting at or below the waist, in the legs, or at all throughout your midsection. Anticipating your belly will grow larger as the weeks and months progress, keep in mind that the snug clothes you purchase this week could be downright tight by next week!

CHAPTER 10

Swimming

Swimming is probably one of the best exercises a pregnant woman can do. Not only is it a great workout, but the buoyancy of the water can help alleviate many problems (such as overheating and jarring movements) associated with exercise and pregnancy. Pregnant women also report feeling great being in the water.

Benefits for Mom and Baby

Swimming is a favorite form of exercise for pregnant women for a variety of reasons. It provides you with a great cardiovascular workout and exercises the majority of your muscle groups. Many women enjoy the feeling of floating and taking stress off their bones and joints. Others enjoy the cool feeling they have while in the pool, even during the colder months. Some just find the water relaxing.

Overall, swimming is an excellent way to stay physically and mentally fit during your pregnancy. Swimming also offers the added benefit of being readily available to all fitness levels.

FACT

When you're in water, you feel much lighter than on the land. For example, 150 pounds feels like it weighs about 15 pounds while submerged. This feels great when you're sporting the extra pounds of pregnancy!

Open to All

Swimming is one of the few exercises that you can do during pregnancy, even if you have not been a frequent exerciser prior to pregnancy. This is good news for you if you've not previously been swimming, or if your overall fitness level is not as high as you'd like it to be. You can start by swimming easily for twenty minutes a day. Do this three to four times a week, and feel free to build yourself up to a routine that consists of six to seven swimming sessions per week that last between twenty and forty minutes.

Movement

Being pregnant can cause a variety of weight-related problems, particularly when it comes to your joints and bones. While in water, you feel lighter and do not have as many concerns with the bumping and jarring of being on land. The more pregnant you become, the more relaxin (a hormone secreted by the placenta and the lining of the uterus) your body releases. While this is of great benefit during labor, when you want your pelvis to move more freely, it can cause a variety of aches and pains during pregnancy.

The buoyancy of the water allows you to move around freely. Many pregnant women report to be more limber while in water. This beneficial aspect can help make your workout easier, not to mention its effect on pain relief! Buoyancy also helps protect you from injury due to exercise.

Posture Aid

Being in the pool also aids with your posture. It's easier to be upright in the pool. Maintaining proper positioning of your body will help alleviate and prevent some problems associated with pregnancy. The water also acts as a massage agent by exerting force on your body and massaging your muscles as you move around.

Being in the water does require some balance. This is something you may struggle with during pregnancy. However, in the water you're not as likely to fall and injure yourself as you may be on land. This adds difficulty to the workout while still allowing you to exercise your balance and work on improvements.

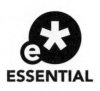

ESSENTIAL

You can also use the buoyancy of the water to provide resistance for your workouts. Using the water to ease your workouts and increase the difficulty can take some time, so just get used to the feel of the water first, if you're not used to exercising in the aquatic environment.

Relaxation

Just as when you were a kid, swimming or even being in water can leave you physically exhausted. While you may feel exhausted on a general basis, this form of exhaustion and relaxation is more conducive to sleeping than general pregnancy exhaustion.

We know that exercising helps pregnant women and others get more rest at night. Exercising in water has this same benefit. In addition, exercise in water offers the added benefit of feeling less weighed down by the added weight of pregnancy; others are simply more relaxed in water.

Blood Pressure

Ah, here's a great benefit that many people do not know about. If you have blood pressure problems, particularly while pregnant, simply being in shoulder-deep water can help decrease your overall blood pressure. This is due to increased circulation and relief from swelling. There is also a decrease in the associated risks of high blood pressure.

Where to Swim

Finding the time to exercise is always talked about, but what about finding a place to swim? Many people are lucky enough to have indoor pools located fairly close to their homes. And the majority of us know where to swim in the summer. However, choosing a place to swim for exercise might be a completely different task than swimming with the kids.

You will want to find a place that has not only convenient hours and locations, but also fees that are reasonable. Many locations offer swim-only memberships. Some natatoriums offer discounts if you take their classes. Be sure to check out the prices and availability. Nothing is more frustrating than going to swim to find the lap lanes filled with a toddler class.

ALERT

Be careful about being out in the sun during pregnancy. In addition to the normal sun-exposure risks, your skin is more sensitive throughout pregnancy. You might be more likely to burn or develop splotches from exposure. Sunscreen will help you protect your pregnant glow without the fear of the splotchy skin.

Check your local YMCA, JCC, and even local colleges for places to swim indoors. Many outdoor pools are also joining the competition and placing bubbles, heated covers, and plastic buildings over their pools to make them accessible in the winter. You might even ask members of local swim clubs for their recommendations for wintertime swimming locations.

Water Exercises

Not everyone will be able to find or attend an organized swimming class or water aerobics session. This doesn't mean that you can't benefit from water aerobics as a form of pregnancy exercise. Simply find your own workout for the pool.

The Lap Lane

For the experienced swimmer, the lap lane is the place where it all happens. You get your lane and you go. This can be a very wonderful form of exercise. It allows you to set the pace and control how far you go. As you progress in pregnancy, you may find that you have no trouble maintaining your normal lap schedule. If you do need to cut back either in distance or speed, they are easily adjusted.

ALERT

When swimming, be sure to watch your form. Kicking too vigorously has the potential to injure your pubic symphysis because of the added hormone relaxin. Flutter kicking is fine, as is moderate breaststroke kicking; just don't overdo it.

Be sure you know the rules of your lap pool. Is there a certain way to turn around? If it involves going underwater, are you okay with that? What about which direction you swim in? Some pools have alternating directions. Will you be expected to share lanes? Is there a time limit to how long you can have a lane? Be sure you know these rules of the pool before you jump in.

Pool Walking

By breathing naturally and walking around the pool as you would on the ground, you can get some good exercise. This is called "traveling in the pool." You can do other exercises and then spend a few minutes walking around the pool. Over the course of your workout you will accumulate this traveling time into a workout of its own. This is best done in shallow water, no higher than waist deep.

Pool Jogging

Unlike regular jogging, which can be jarring to the system, running in water offers you some padding. It is often used to help runners rehabilitate after an injury, or surgery, as an acceptable form of running.

The basics are the same as for running outside the pool. You can even wear your running shoes, though they are not necessary. You can run in place or move around in a small area of the pool.

For an added workout, add your arms while you run. If this is too much work, you can always stop the arm movements. Remember to warm up and cool down, even in the pool.

FACT

Just moving in the water takes more energy than moving outside the pool. The resistance from the water is what helps provide you with the workout. So if you find yourself in the pool, just move around and see how you start to feel. With a bit of coordination, it's a complete workout!

Hanging On to the Edge

The edge of the pool is a great place to work out. This is particularly true if you're concerned about floating away, or if you're not incredibly tall.

Go to the edge of the pool and hang on to the lip of the pool. Be sure to avoid the areas where there are drains or stairs. These will be more dangerous and high traffic areas.

Hang on and just start moving. It doesn't matter if you face in or out. Try some simple flutters with your feet. You can advance to more full-fledged kicking as you feel you are able to do so. This will provide you with a safe and quiet workout without leaving the pool.

Treading Water

While you might believe it to be just child's play or something done to prove you won't drown yourself, treading water is a great workout. The movement of your arms and legs will keep you afloat but also provide you with a lot of exercise for two large muscle groups.

Your legs aren't what you want to move? Try doing some basic arm movements, like circles. Alternate big circles with small circles. Go forward and backward in direction. Hold your arms in front of your chest with your arms bent in and twist slowly at the waist.

ESSENTIAL

Chlorine exposure is minimal while swimming, but for added safety and to decrease potential exposure, always end your workout session with a shower to rinse off any chemicals from the pool. This is good advice for any swimmer.

Even bouncing up and down while making splashing movements with your arms can be fun and a good workout. For some added workout, try to propel yourself out of the pool, like a rocket. First, bend your knees slightly and then push up with your feet while you push down with your arms. Even kids can get into this exercise.

Water Aerobics

Water aerobics is great fun! Many gyms and fitness centers now offer water aerobics as a part of their programs. Some even specifically have pregnancy water aerobics. While it is not necessary to find a class that is specifically geared toward pregnancy, it is imperative that you talk to the instructor about your pregnancy. This allows him or her to alert you to changes you need to make while participating in the class.

Exercise Aids

While swimming or doing water aerobics, some pregnant women desire using some of the varied exercise aids. These can include water weights, flotation devices, and so forth.

You might consider using them to help you exercise or to help you relax. Many moms resort to using flotation devices in the final months of pregnancy. This allows more of your body to remain underwater, while allowing you to float, much like your baby floats.

Kick boards are another water aid that can be useful while pregnant. Try taking a kick board with you as you semi-float around the pool. It can be useful to lie your head on as you float, or you can use it to hang on to while kicking your legs away.

A deep-water flotation belt can be handy if you aren't the best swimmer or you are trying to do your workouts in the deep end. The problem is that by the end of the second trimester, the belt may not fit your growing abdomen. Exercise caution when in deep water and talk to the lifeguards and other pool personnel about the use of flotation belts.

The Necessary Precautions

Exercising in water can be very deceptive—you get a great workout with what feels like less effort, but feeling less intensity during your workout can lead you to become overheated, overexerted, or dehydrated if you're not paying close attention to your body's needs. Submerged in the water, the body can maintain a comfortable temperature and muscles can feel less strained, but the lessened limitations come with the need for added attention to the length or duration of your workout, adequately hydrating before, during, and after, and being aware of any and all signs of discomfort that could signal improper form during exercise or overuse of certain muscles. You can avoid the "danger zone" of swimming by simply drinking more than enough water (keeping in mind that thirst is a sign of dehydration) and listening to your body; remember that your regular exercise is intended to help, not hurt!

FACT

Water temperature is very important in pregnancy. Most pools keep their water temperature between 82 and 86 degrees Fahrenheit. This temperature level is fine for pregnant women. Be sure to see where the water temperature of your pool is posted and check it daily to ensure it's within a healthy range for your swim.

Here are a few warning signs that exercise in water would *not* be appropriate:

- If your amniotic sac, or bag of water, was broken or leaking
- If you had an infection
- If you were experiencing preterm labor or another contraindication to exercise

Simple Stretches and Exercises for the Pool

Whether you're looking to stretch, strengthen, or tone, there are a couple quick and easy exercises you can perform in the pool to do just that! From squats, lunges, and leg lifts to your laps or free-style swim, you can enjoy a well-rounded workout that boasts cardiovascular benefits as well as benefits to the muscles in your legs, butt, and back.

Squatting

Go to the water level that is chest deep for you. Place your feet about hip-width apart and keep your toes pointing forward. Sit back with your bottom and allow your arms to come up to the front, chest level for balance. Push yourself back to the original pose using your feet, while bringing your arms to the sides. This can be a very easy exercise. To make it harder, try doing it in more shallow water. Remember, squats help prepare your body for birth. The repetitive strengthening of the leg muscles helps you assume positions of birth to make it faster and easier for you. Try this exercise for eight to ten repetitions.

Lunges

In chest-deep water, stand with your feet hip-width apart. Take a step backward, placing your weight between the sole of the front foot and the ball of your back foot. Bend your knees until you've reached as far as you can go. You should not go lower than is comfortable or so low that your neck is underwater. Hold the pose for a few seconds and then push up to your original pose. You can alternate feet or do one side at a time. You should do eight to ten repetitions of this exercise for full benefit. Again, to increase the difficulty of this exercise, try doing it in more shallow water.

Leg Lifts

This is another simple exercise you can do while in the pool. In chest-deep water, stand with your feet hip-width apart. Stand with soft knees and bring your left leg up toward the surface, toes pointed up. Go as far as you can without losing balance or injuring yourself. Repeat this eight to ten times and then switch legs.

CHAPTER 11

Yoga

The use of yoga during pregnancy may be the perfect combination of exercise, centering, and relaxation. Not only will this exercise form work out your body, but it will allow you to exercise your mind and help relieve stress as well. It is also easily adapted for all fitness levels, including some women on bed rest or women with exercise restrictions during pregnancy.

Prenatal Yoga

Yoga is derived from the Sanskrit word *yuk*, which means "yoke," or to join together. The basic translation has come to be "union." Using the concept of the union of body, mind, and soul, yoga offers many benefits to you during your pregnancy, birth, and postpartum. Some practitioners look at it as a bonding of mother and baby, even before birth.

The benefits of yoga go beyond the typical benefits of the physical body. Yoga is definitely a fitness activity that takes the mind and soul into consideration as well. This can be very useful to you throughout pregnancy, as well as months down the road when you begin your journey into parenthood, even if it is not the first time you have been down this path.

Yoga is actually a generic term used to encompass many different forms of yoga. Hatha yoga, Iyengar yoga, and ashtanga yoga are the most common forms in the Western world. But there are many more forms of yoga. Each of these forms employs an ancient concept of physical well-being and balance with the mental and spiritual side of your body and soul. They stress strength, relaxation, and flexibility as a way to unite the body. Over the years, prenatal yoga has become a specific form of the practice that focuses on the poses and holds that promote healthy body, mind, and relaxation techniques for each trimester of pregnancy.

By using poses, or *asanas*, you learn to strengthen your body, increase your flexibility, and develop a sense of inner wisdom and peace as you learn more about your pregnant body.

Strengthening

When you begin to challenge your body with yoga's movements, positions, and strategic holds, you'll be challenging your body to perform in ways that it simply doesn't on a regular basis. From poses that stretch your muscles to holds that require your muscles to maintain a particular position for a couple of seconds, your body's muscles will become stronger and work more efficiently. As you progress from a beginner to a more advanced yoga participant, you'll notice that the movements that were challenging to begin with no longer require as much effort. This progression is great for your body because it means your muscles are beginning to work better with one another in order to perform, in addition to getting stronger as they deal with the workload of the new challenges that are posed with more experienced practice.

All of the strengthening that occurs throughout the body will help you maintain better posture throughout your pregnancy, helping to alleviate discomfort and minimize injuries. In addition to posture improvement throughout pregnancy, you can look forward to the benefits of greater strength and flexibility and improved muscle control during labor and delivery. Following the birth of your baby, you'll likely be one of the women who reports faster healing time and enjoys improved strength as you begin toting around your infant well into the toddler years!

Stress Reduction

Stress is something that has a negative effect on your life. Yoga has been used for centuries to help reduce the amount of stress felt by an individual. Pregnancy creates stressors that you may not anticipate, even if this is a much-planned pregnancy. Yoga accomplishes this stress reduction with a few simple techniques: centering, breathing, and poses.

Centering

Centering is a way of getting in touch with your body. Through a combination of breathing, poses, and centering, you will learn techniques to help you and your body through pregnancy. Often this component of yoga is referred to as meditation.

Meditation requires practice and skill. It is not something that comes automatically to many people. During pregnancy, learning the ability to put other thoughts out of your mind and to focus on your body and your baby will have many benefits.

Breathing

Say the word *breathing* to nearly any pregnant woman and her mind immediately goes to the old patterned paced breathing, often associated with panting dogs and laboring women. Not only is this form of breathing not appropriate for labor and birth, it's not great for pregnant women either. Breathing in yoga is a completely different form.

Ujayi breathing, or the yoga breath, is said to promote calmness and a feeling of well-being. During your pregnancy, practicing this form of breathing can be beneficial to you and your baby in many ways. It will help you learn relaxation techniques that are beneficial for labor. As your mind and body relax, you are better able to give birth with reduced amounts of pain.

ALERT

To master yoga breathing, you will need to practice. Start by breathing deeply through your mouth. Begin to make a silent "ha," as if you're fogging up a mirror. Now, do the same as you inhale. (You'll see why it's called "ocean breath.") Once you're comfortable with the technique, close your mouth and breathe through your nose.

You can add thoughts to the breathing as well. For example, imagine as you breathe in that you are bringing good, clean air to your baby. "See" that breath travel down through your body and through the placenta and umbilical cord to your baby. Then as you exhale, imagine carrying away all the toxins in your body, away from your baby.

FACT

Breathing is a well-known way to reduce stress and to increase relaxation. This is the foundation of most childbirth classes. What type of breathing is practiced varies from organization to organization. Be sure to ask your potential teachers which form of breathing they use.

Learning to control your breath is also important in the pushing phase of labor. Doing yoga-type breathing during this phase will increase your oxygen levels as well as those of your baby. This makes it safer and more satisfying for you as you push your baby into this world.

Focus

It is also important to note that yoga is process-oriented rather than goal-oriented. This means it does not matter how many times you perform a movement or pose, but that you focus on it while participating fully. Tackle each pose as if it is the only pose you will do. Focus completely and entirely on the pose as you do it. Do not let your mind wander to the next pose or the day ahead, because your focus should consistently remain on your form throughout any pose. This is a different viewpoint from regular exercise that frequently focuses on the number of repetitions.

Remember—when doing poses, never do them to the point of exhaustion. Never bend or stretch further than is comfortable. And hold them only as long as you feel steady and relaxed.

Best Prenatal Poses

There are many poses involved in yoga. Many of these poses are perfectly appropriate for pregnancy. Using them alone or in conjunction with other forms of exercise can greatly enhance your skills and preparation.

Child's Pose

Kneel on the floor, separating your knees slightly. Put your big toes together and sit back with your buttocks on the heels of your feet. Stretch your arms over your head. Hold this pose for five seconds, releasing a bit more with each breath. If this reach is too far for you as a beginner or later in pregnancy, bend your elbows and rest on your forearms to alleviate some of the tension.

Forward Bend

Stand with your feet as wide apart as is comfortable. Lean forward onto two supports to hold your body weight. Focus on keeping your chest open. Hold your head up to allow a good stretch of your neck.

Modified Forward Bend

To open the pelvic area, sit on the floor with your thighs spread apart to accommodate your growing abdomen. Bend forward at the back and hold your toes with your hands if you can. Keep the knees straight.

Cat Balance

While kneeling on the floor, pull in your abdominal muscles and breathe naturally. As you exhale, extend your right leg and left arm. Think about extending each limb as far as you comfortably can. Hold this pose for three to five breaths. Repeat ten times on each side.

Modified Cobra Pose

Stand with feet together, or separated if that is more comfortable, with your hands clasped behind your back. Inhale and drop your head back. Hold this pose and breathe gently. Inhale again, arching your back while pushing your chest out and your arms back. Finally, push your hips forward. This can avoid abdominal pressure and strengthen the legs while giving your back a good stretch and backward bend.

Wall Butterfly

Lie down on the floor with your bottom and feet against the wall, keep your soles together, and let your knees drop open. Use your hands to press your knees downward toward the wall. This exercise will open up your pelvic area. It also helps to strengthen your legs, inner thighs, and lower spine.

You can also do this pose seated with a partner. Simply sit and pull your knees up as close as is comfortable to your body. Have your partner hold your outer legs at about knee level. Have him or her provide slight resistance as you try to separate your legs. This is a great way to get others involved in your pregnancy! Even a school-aged child can help here.

Wall Squat

Standing up straight with your back facing a wall, place the birth ball (a "yoga ball" or "exercise ball" that can be purchased at sports stores or most stores that have a sports section) between you and the wall around the center of your back and press it into the wall using your back. Slowly walk your feet forward, leaning back into the ball for support. As you walk forward, the ball will roll up to the center of your back, between your shoulder blades. This allows you to do a squat without having to worry about being steady or having a partner for added support. Once you are down as far as you can go without your knees approaching your toes, hold the pose for up to ten seconds, and then slowly walk your feet back to their starting position, allowing the ball to roll back to the center of your lower back.

Down Dog

This is not a beginner pose. Stand with your feet hip-width apart. Bend at the hips over a collection of supports or a chair. This can be a stack of towels or blankets over a bed, or anything about waist height. Rest your hands and your arms on the supports in front of you. Your head will probably be about thigh level, depending on your flexibility. If your heels come up off the floor, have someone place supports under your feet. You may require help getting into this pose.

What *Not* to Do

Although yoga is a great form of exercise for pregnancy, there are a few precautions you must remember. The first thing to remember is that above all else, if anything hurts—stop. This is a basic rule of exercise during pregnancy. You may tend to forget about yoga as a form of exercise, but these basics still hold true.

Pregnancy is an acceptable time to start yoga, even if you have never done it before. Some instructors advise that you wait until you are in the second trimester to begin yoga if you have never done it before. However, in the absence of any medical indications not to exercise, yoga is perfectly acceptable in the first trimester. Always let your instructor know you are expecting.

ESSENTIAL

Remember to give your baby room as you are doing poses. If you need to modify a pose to fit your expanding abdomen, simply try spreading your legs a bit wider, although you do need to focus on balance as well.

Remember that your body is full of hormones, including relaxin. This will cause you to be more susceptible to injury, including overstretching.

Listen to your body. It will provide you with signals that you are going too far. Use towels and bands to help you reach your feet in certain poses.

When bending, remember to bend at the back, not at your hips. This will be more comfortable on your body. Keeping your upper back as straight as possible will also help decrease discomfort and breathing difficulties. In a seated position, use the towel around your feet to help you remain upright.

Balance Issues

Many poses in yoga will require balance. This is something you don't have a lot of while pregnant. Try to do these poses near the wall or a chair to help you maintain your balance, particularly after the fourth month. If this is not possible, skip these poses and save them for postpartum use.

Poses that require you to lie on your back or stomach should be avoided after about four months of pregnancy. If you find they are uncomfortable sooner, discontinue them at that point. Don't wait until a certain arbitrary time. Always use good judgment while doing any form of exercise. Remember, listen to your body.

Your Kind of Yoga

Yoga does not have to be done in a classroom, nor does it have to be done alone. There are a variety of ways to approach your yoga education.

FACT

While other exercise classes offer teachers with certification, there is no such thing as a national or international certification for a yoga instructor. This is partially because there are many forms of yoga and many different organizations. Look for an instructor with a long history of teaching. Ask to speak to other students in the class for their opinion.

Yoga Classes

There are plenty of yoga classes available in most cities. There are also more and more classes for pregnancy yoga. To find out what is available where you live, try looking up yoga in the phone book and calling some different centers.

If they do offer yoga classes specifically for pregnancy, ask about the class population. Is it made up of beginners? Or are a variety of levels taught in one class? Does the instructor have any specific pregnancy-related credentials?

Classes are nice because they offer a built-in support system and an instructor who can answer questions and make suggestions. If the class is composed of other pregnant women, it can really be helpful that you are all experiencing similar life changes. But classes are not necessary for the success of your yoga program.

Yoga Videos

Yoga videos can be another great way to experience yoga during pregnancy. There are many forms of yoga classes available on DVD from a wide variety of instructors. Always try to get a reference for a good video from a yoga practitioner or even reviews of videos. This can prevent you from going through several videos trying to find the right fit.

ALERT

When doing yoga on your own, make sure you choose a well-ventilated room for your practice sessions. Level flooring is also important to your balance issues. Bring any props you will need, such as a mat, strap, or blanket. The room should be free of distractions, drafts, and moisture.

Yoga Books

There are many yoga books with sections on pregnancy and yoga. There are also quite a few yoga books specifically designed for pregnant women. Look for books with clear instructions and photos to help you. Also ask around to see what books others are using.

CHAPTER 12

Fabulous Arms

During pregnancy, many women tend to focus on their abdomen, legs, and maybe their back. However, one of the most often neglected areas is the arms. Learning to exercise this part of your body is simple and not very time-consuming, but the benefits are great!

Muscles

When you think of your arms, you might immediately think of how they look in sleeveless dresses, or you might think of strength issues. But truth be told, many people neglect their arms and pregnant women are no different. Let's look at the different areas of the arm, how they work, and what you can do to make the most out of your arm muscles for fitness and fashion.

Chest Muscles

Women aren't often thought of as having chest muscles. But you do! A woman's chest muscles are simply covered with the breast tissue that helps her nurture her children after birth. The chest muscles are composed of two muscles: pectoralis major and pectoralis minor.

The pectoralis major is a fan-shaped muscle near the surface that runs horizontally from the middle of your clavicle, or collarbone, to your upper arm. It also encompasses the area from your sternum, or breastbone, diagonally to the upper arm. This muscle helps you move your arms upward, inward, and across your body.

Working out your chest muscles will not cause you to bulk up. While you will have firmer muscles under your breasts, very few women look like the typical bodybuilder. This will also not significantly change the shape of your breasts, nor interfere with breastfeeding.

ESSENTIAL

Stretching, particularly before and after feeding your baby, will help release tension in your arms and back. Massage is also a great idea. It's a great way to pamper the new mom, but is also very good for releasing that tension. This can be done by anyone, including a professional masseur or masseuse.

Biceps and Triceps

When you think of arm muscles, the two that are most prominent are the triceps and the biceps, the main muscles in your arms. There are other muscles involved in working out your arms, but focusing on the biceps and triceps will ensure that all these muscles are worked as well.

When working out your arms, it is important to remember to work both the biceps in the front and the triceps in the back equally. If you fail to do this, the muscles are going to develop differently, causing you problems down the road. These muscles work together in an important fashion. Think about bending your arm at the elbow, as your biceps contract to bend the elbow. What happens to the triceps in the rear of your arm? The triceps naturally stretch. This give and take is an important balance to visualize and understand.

Back and Shoulder Muscles

While you might not think of these muscles as being part of your arms, the shoulder and back muscles are primary movement makers of your arms. Keeping them strong and healthy will help you with your arm movements and strength. Your back muscles also include the latissimus dorsi, the trapezius muscles, and the rhomboid muscles.

These muscles also assist in holding your body erect. They provide support and will help in nursing your baby. Often, a good massage of the upper back before or after a nursing session will be helpful and will feel great.

ALERT

When working your arms, you need to be sure that you are not extending your arms forcefully or completely. This can actually injure your arm muscles. When doing your exercises, remember to stop just short of a full extension and to use smooth movements to prevent injury.

Forearms

Your forearms are important to pay attention to as well, though we usually forget this portion of the body very quickly. After all, what do the forearms really do for you? They do plenty. The strength of your forearms determines how strong your grip will be, provides stabilization for your wrists, and provides you with protection from injury of the arm and hand.

Stretching the forearm can be very important, particularly if you use your hands or wrists much in computer work, perform fine motor skills with your hands, or simply while feeding your baby. The forearms will bear the brunt of all of your arm work.

Hands

Some of the more frequent problems pregnant women experience in their hands are carpal tunnel syndrome and repetitive motion syndrome. Both of these problems are more common in pregnancy. The reason you will see these flare up during pregnancy is because of the added swelling of your tissues.

You may notice a tingling sensation or numbness in your hands and fingers. This can be particularly bad if you work with your hands. If you type a lot at the computer, you are particularly at risk for suffering during pregnancy. If you work at a job where you do the same repetitive motion over and over, then you are also at risk for one of these problems.

However, the good news is that, most of the time, birth will help cure some of your problems with carpal tunnel and repetitive motion syndromes. This is because your body fluid levels will go back to your pre-pregnancy state and relieve some of the added swelling on nerves and the like in your arms and hands. Obviously, if it flares up during pregnancy, you can expect to see it again later in life, during another pregnancy or just as you naturally age.

How to Prevent Injuries

There are a couple of simple solutions and exercises that you can try to prevent carpal tunnel and repetitive motion syndromes from becoming problems. These exercises and strategies also work in helping to alleviate any pain you are already experiencing.

Inspect your workstation by looking around at what is at your desk and how everything is set up. Do you practice good ergonomics? Are you too far away from your keyboard or desk? Ideally, you should be able to keep your arms and elbows relatively close to your body.

Wrist and Hand Protectors

Your wrists should be supported at the keyboard. This can be by using a wrist pad made of several different materials, including gel pads. This prevents your wrists from being lower than your hands and allows for better circulation and relaxation. You should also have a pad at your mouse.

Wrist splints are also helpful in alleviating pain and complications, although they can be uncomfortable to wear. You can purchase hand/wrist splints at most drug stores and physical therapy centers. Many doctors can also prescribe splints that are specifically made to fit your arms. You will probably be able to wear these only at night, as they prevent you from cutting off circulation to your hands during sleep by bending your wrists or sleeping with your hands in funny positions.

Benefits of Arm Exercises

Most of the exercises you do in pregnancy seem to be geared toward something to help directly with your pregnancy and well-being. However, it is the arms that you really need to focus on, since you use this area of your body all the time but with very little thought. The good news is that very few complications of pregnancy preclude your arm exercises.

Your arms will be used somewhat in labor, particularly during the pushing phase. You will use them to help pull your legs back or to hold your body up as you push. This can be very tiring if your arms are not used to working out. However, remember that at the end of your hard work, a miracle is placed in these same arms—your baby.

While the work of labor might seem to be enough of a reason to exercise your arms during your pregnancy, there are others. Postpartum is probably the biggest reason to exercise your arms.

During the postpartum phase, having strong arms is very important. Your arms will be carrying around your new baby and strong arms make that task much easier to bear. Your forearms and wrists will be used repeatedly during the day as you feed, change, and bathe your baby. There is no area of the arm that is not used in daily baby care. And that doesn't even mention mom care!

Tools

If you want to start an exercise routine that includes arm-focused exercises, there are a couple of tools you could use to maximize your exercise benefits. Although the list includes some items that you may already own, note that there is no need to buy or use any of these unless you feel they would make for a more beneficial workout.

- **Dumbbells:** Weights that range between 2 and 8 pounds would offer a light to moderately difficult workout that could vary depending upon your choosing.
- **Resistance Bands:** As an alternative to weights, you could use resistance bands that add an element of resistance to movements that would be far less difficult without them.
- **Mat:** Having a supportive mat that provides cushioning and traction while you're working out is essential to ensure that you remain safe and supported while performing your exercises.

Using Weights for Arm Work

While weights are definitely not an absolute necessity, they can be very helpful in your arm fitness program. Simple resistance may not be enough for some women, and this might be especially true for you if you've had a lot of exercise experience with your arms.

If you are more advanced in your arm work, bands might be only a temporary solution as you are getting back into your regular routine or if your pregnancy calls for cutting back on certain exercises.

ESSENTIAL

Avoid dropping your weights on the floor after use. You should set them down gently. This will not only avoid injuring yourself but will keep your equipment lasting longer.

There is not one weight that is right or wrong for everyone. The best test of weight limit is your comfort level. Lifting weights should be a slight strain, but it should never feel overpowering. Lifting too much weight can damage your muscles, so watching what you lift is important. Increase your weights gradually. Consider a personal training meeting if you have significant questions about weights.

Sample Arm-Specific Exercises

Exercises that work your arms, back, and shoulders can help you in your every-day life. Many are simple and require only a few repetitions to be effective.

Biceps Curl

Stand with soft knees shoulder-width apart. Pull in your abdominal muscles and lift your chest. Remember to keep your spine elongated. Tuck your elbows into your sides, forearms facing upward. Close your fists and slowly raise your fist to your chest. You can do this one arm at a time or two at a time. You should use your body as resistance at first. Do this exercise ten times on each side to work your biceps. As you get stronger, you can add hand weights or dumbbells to increase resistance.

FACT

The average full-term baby will weigh about 7½ pounds at birth. While this sounds like a very little weight to have to carry around, the truth is that carrying around 7-plus pounds for more than about thirty minutes will cause your arms and back to ache and become very sore. Strong muscles will help alleviate this problem.

Alternate Biceps Curls

Stand with your feet shoulder-width apart and pointing forward so that you have a solid base. Take a weight and place it in your left hand. Keep your left elbow close to your side, with your arm bent parallel to the floor. Slowly raise the weight to about shoulder level. Slowly lower the weight to the starting position. Do not go too quickly or use jerky movements. If you find yourself struggling or straining, use less weight. Repeat this exercise for eight to ten repetitions. Repeat on the opposite side. You can also do this in a seated position or without weights.

Triceps Pump

Stand with feet shoulder-width apart. With soft knees, bend slightly at the waist with a straight back and gaze forward. Hold weights, bands, or just clenched fists at sides, and push the hands backward until arms are fully extended behind. Return to starting position. Repeat ten times for one set, and perform three sets.

Single Arm Lifts

Stand with one foot slightly forward, and your feet about shoulder-width apart. Stand on your flex band with your right foot, while grasping the other end of the band with your right hand. Palm facing down, slowly raise the right arm to shoulder level. Hold this pose for up to five seconds and slowly lower the right arm. Repeat this motion ten times. Then switch to your left arm for another ten repetitions. As an alternative exercise that works the antagonistic muscles, perform the same exercise, except with palms facing up.

Double Arm Lifts

Stand in the middle of your flex band. Hold one end of the band in each hand, while your arms hang by your sides. Relax and bend your knees slightly, while maintaining your spine in an upright position. Slowly, and together, raise both hands to your sides, palms upward, until you reach shoulder level. Be careful to use only your arms and not your shoulders in this exercise. The goal is to strengthen your arms to help you gain strength for tasks such as lifting your new baby. Do this exercise for ten repetitions.

Side Arm Stretches

Stand with your feet shoulder-width apart. Take the flex band in both hands, with your palms facing upward. Your arms and elbows should be tucked into your sides. Hold the right hand steady as you move your left forearm and hand slowly away from your body. When you reach your limit, slowly bring your left hand back to its starting position. Repeat this exercise ten times. Switch to exercising your right hand, while your left hand remains steady. Do another set of ten repetitions on that side.

Arm Raise Stretch

While seated or standing, inhale and bring your arms over your head, keeping your elbows slightly bent. As you raise your arms, feel your spine loosen and lengthen. As you reach the peak, slowly straighten your elbows with your palms toward the ceiling. Hold this pose for a few seconds and release slowly as you exhale. To steady yourself, try clasping your hands above your head. If your fingers or wrists feel stiff after doing this exercise, shake them very gently to release tension. Repeat this movement often to help release tension.

Lat Stretch

Sit on the floor with a prop or blanket between your legs, supporting your weight. Raise your right arm over your head, and bend it down toward your spine, behind your head. Stretch your fingers downward without straining. Allow the left arm to come up and hold your right elbow. Without pulling, gently stretch the right arm toward the ceiling. Hold this pose for a count of five. This movement should not be bouncy or jerky, as this can hurt your arms. Repeat with your left arm. You may repeat this movement as often as you like.

Kneeling Shoulder Stretch

Kneel on a soft surface on the floor facing a wall (use a towel if you need to), about a foot away from the wall. Spread your knees as far apart as you need to in order to allow your growing belly to rest comfortably on the floor. Turn your feet in toward the center, and drop the lower part of your pelvis, relaxing your pelvic floor as you do. Raise your arms over your head with your palms facing the wall. Place your hands as high above your head on the wall as you can go without straining or causing yourself pain. Consciously think of elongating your spine and relaxing backward onto your feet. Hold this stretch for ten seconds or more. Then release your arms slowly to your side and let your weight rest farther back on your feet. Let your head gently lean forward and feel the stretch between your shoulder blades and in your upper arms.

Wall Pushups

Facing the wall, place your hands palm down on the wall and walk your feet backward, away from the wall. Slowly bend your elbows, bringing your upper body closer to the wall. Do about ten repetitions of the exercise. Remember to keep your spine in the proper alignment while doing this exercise.

Seated Pectoral Stretch

While sitting erect on the floor or on a birth ball, place your hands on your lower back above your buttocks. Concentrate on pulling your shoulder blades together and continue breathing. Do this exercise ten times.

Posture Retraining

Place your back against the wall; slowly walk your feet forward until they are 6 to 8 inches in front of you. Press your glutes, shoulder blades, and the back of your head into the wall. Slowly raise your arms at a 90-degree angle, bent elbow to the wall, and press them to the wall as well. Slowly raise your arms, keeping them on the wall, above your head.

Chest Stretch

Stand with your feet hip-width apart. Take a step forward on either foot. As you inhale, extend your arms to your sides; the palms should be facing forward. Gently stretch back until you feel tension in your chest. If the intensity is too much or you are on bed rest, try doing this exercise in a chair or in your bed. Do several repetitions to help stretch the chest area.

Developing a Program of Exercises

What exercises you choose to do will help develop your muscles. Choosing them will depend on where you are starting at from a strength, flexibility, and tone standpoint. Do not be influenced by what others think you should be doing. Your arms will follow when you lead.

Look for areas that need your attention. Focus on where you have pain or tightness. Sometimes you go for the weak spots. The most important thing is a well-rounded workout for your arms. You don't want to over-exercise certain parts while neglecting others. This can lead to more pain and trouble than you had to begin with! Always balance your arm work.

CHAPTER 13

Awesome Abs (and Back!)

Pregnancy is obviously not the time to worry about a washboard stomach. Your six-pack abs will have to wait until after the birth of your baby. With that said, there is still plenty that you can do to work your abdominal muscles during pregnancy without going overboard or injuring yourself.

Muscles

Your abdominal muscles run from under your breastbone all the way to your pubic bone. This set of muscles is called the *rectus abdominis*. Underneath the rectus muscles are two sets of muscles that run at an angle toward the center of your abdomen, called your *obliques*. These muscles help you twist and turn and define your waist. The layer beneath the obliques is called the *transversus abdominis*. Running the entire length of your abdomen, this muscle supports your organs. It also covers a lot of area under your other muscles.

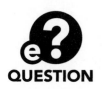

QUESTION

Is a pre-pregnancy "six-pack" going to keep my body from changing as it should?
If you have great abs prior to pregnancy, you may worry that your six-pack will prevent your body from growing and expanding as it should. It is important to note that this is not the case, and your baby will grow just fine. Be sure to check with your practitioner at every visit for an update of your uterine growth.

Benefits of Strong Abdominal Muscles

Popular literature used to say that you should never exercise your abdominal muscles during pregnancy because of a fear that it would harm your pregnancy or your baby. Today, we realize that these muscles are so important for pregnancy and beyond that we have had to rethink our teachings about abdominal exercise in pregnancy. The consensus is now that while it is safe to exercise your abdominal muscles during pregnancy, certain precautions must be taken.

Abs in Birth and Beyond

You might wonder why we bother talking about abdominal muscles during pregnancy if the benefits can't be seen or, supposedly, used during pregnancy. The reason you should be exercising these muscles is that they are being used on a daily basis, regardless of whether or not you are consciously working them. Poor muscle tone in this area can lead to increased pregnancy complaints and weakness that can result in poor posture and back pain long after your pregnancy.

Back pain is one of the most common complaints of pregnancy. The surprising fact is that much of your back pain can have to do with your abdominal muscles. How strong and toned your abs are will dictate how well your back is supported. This is not to say that abdominal work is all you need to prevent back pain, but having an imbalance of either set of your muscles will contribute to your pain and discomfort.

Assessing Your Abdominal Needs

Before any abdominal workout in pregnancy, it is important to know where you're starting from. If you had great abdominal muscles prior to pregnancy, you may worry about the loss of tone or definition. While it is true that your waist and abdomen do disappear during pregnancy, the muscles that you have attained are able to maintain tone and fitness, while providing you with a stable body.

If you've never really given your abdominal muscles much thought, now might be the time to start. An important first step is to recognize any problems you currently have with your abdominal muscles.

Diastasis Recti

It is highly recommended that you check your rectus muscles along the central seam, directly down the center of your abdominal muscle, for a separation, known as diastasis recti. This condition can occur for many reasons, pregnancy being one of them. However, you can work on this diastasis recti during pregnancy to help lessen its effects and decrease the width.

No matter what anyone tells you, the truth is that there is no cure or absolute prevention for stretch marks. A well-toned body, good nutritional status, and well-hydrated skin all help in the fight against stretch marks, although genetics will win every time. Avoid the magic cures that promise miracle cures or prevention treatment.

To check for the diastasis recti, begin by lying on your back with your knees bent. Slowly raise your head and shoulders, stretching your arms toward your knees. Place the fingers of one hand horizontally just above your belly button, in the center, near the seam of your muscles. You will know you are in the right spot because you can feel the abdominal muscles tighten on each side. Make note of how many fingers fit in this area of separation. A large separation would indicate that your focus needs to be on proper form during exercise, and keeping in mind that any activity you do flat on your back that pulls on your abdominal muscles is going to further that separation.

Limitations and Modifications

When exercising your abdominal muscles, it is important to note that the exercises are most effective on these muscles when you do them while lying on your back. It's not recommended that pregnant women lie flat on their backs for an extended period of time after 16 weeks. Therefore, do your abdominal work in other positions, including all fours, standing, or sitting.

Know Your Absolute Limits

Your abdominal muscles are so important to your overall health and fitness level that it's absolutely imperative to focus on these muscles during pregnancy and beyond. Including some form of abs work in every workout can be very easy to do. However, remember to be wary of too much exercise or exercises that are too challenging for your stage of pregnancy. No supine abdominal exercises are safe past the first trimester, and most of your abdominal work past the first trimester should consist of side-lying exercises or stretches. Keep in mind that you should never assume a position that is painful or hold a stretch that causes burning, pain, or extreme discomfort.

Exercises

Exercises for your abs may bring to mind hard workouts that leave you gasping for breath. The truth is that even the smallest exercise can have a lasting effect on your abdominal muscles. That said, exercising your abs should always be a part of your workout. There are abdominal exercises that can be done by everyone, including when you are very pregnant or newly postpartum.

Breathing

Your breath and breathing will be a very important key to many things in your pregnancy. Exercise and fitness are only the beginning of the need to be aware of your breath. Do not be tempted to ignore your breathing. It will be the key to relaxation in labor and will help you focus. It will help you to exercise and tone your muscles through appropriate concentration. It also tones your mind as well as your body.

Deep abdominal breathing sounds easy. The good news is that it is very easy. Learning to do true deep abdominal breathing while pregnant is simple, because you've got a great target—your baby. Sit erect with your spine as elongated as possible. Close your eyes and inhale very deeply. Imagine taking the air in and directing it toward your baby. If you have trouble breathing slowly, try counting your breaths. Slowly count to five as you inhale. Hold that breath for several seconds and then slowly release the breath for a count of five.

Modified Oblique Crunch

Lying on your right side, bend your knees slightly so that your knees are in front of your body's midline and your feet are behind your body's midline. With your right hand supporting your head (but not exerting pressure at all), your left arm on your side, and your left hand on your abs, use your obliques to slightly raise your right shoulder off of the floor. With your hand on your abdominals, you should feel tightening on the left side of your stomach, not in the center. If you do feel more of a stretch in the middle of your abs instead of your side, readjust your body until the focus is on the obliques. Remember, you should not feel any discomfort or pain. Perform ten to twelve repetitions for one set.

Abdominal Strengthening

Sit on a birth ball with your feet about hip-distance apart. Sit up on the ball and elongate your spine. You want to keep your spine elongated and pull your abdominal muscles in toward your belly button as you exhale.

If it helps you, imagine coughing to find the abdominal muscles. Breathe normally as you do this exercise. Repeat the exercise ten times. This exercise is appropriate for all phases of pregnancy and recovery. It is also great for beginning relaxation.

Abdominal Tightening

Seated on a birth ball, place your hands on your abdomen. Tilt your pelvis and as you inhale pull your abdominal muscles inward. Feel your abdomen move as your hands rest on them. Hold the pose for five seconds, while breathing. Repeat this exercise ten times.

Kneeling Abdominal Curl

Kneeling on the floor with your hands forward, palms down, tilt your pelvis in, pulling your baby toward the center of your body. Hold this pose for a count of ten. Repeat ten times. You can also do this by leaning across a chair to support your upper body.

Pelvic Rock/Pelvic Tilt

This is a hallmark pregnancy exercise. It provides so many benefits. You will see it mentioned in many categories because of its importance to your health and fitness status. The basic pelvic tilt is done on hands and knees, with your back straight, not sagging. Isolate your pelvis and tilt it toward your abdomen. As you do so, inhale and hold your breath to the count of five. Imagine pulling your abdominal muscles in at your belly button. Slowly release to a neutral position.

Side Bending (Tail Wagging)

This is a great exercise that can also provide you with a stretch. On hands and knees, with your back straight and not sagging, slowly pull your right hip toward your right shoulder. The only part of your body that moves is your hips. Be sure to hold your shoulders and upper body still. Go as far as is comfortable for your body. Repeat this exercise ten times on each side. You can do these exercises one side at a time or alternate one side and then the next. To modify this exercise, try leaning over a chair or a birth ball to support your upper body. This is also a great exercise if you are having side pain.

Abdominals and Labor

You know that your abdominal muscles support your internal organs, and this is true of the uterus as well. Your abdominal muscles will be busy at work during your labor, supporting your uterus as it contracts to open your cervix. By knowing these muscles well, you can help to keep them relaxed. This will help your baby enter your pelvis in a timely and efficient fashion, and therefore actually help speed labor along.

If you are asked not to push for any reason during the second stage of labor, lift your chin from your chest and look upward. Begin to breathe lightly, imagining a feather is floating above your face. Breathe as if to keep that feather from falling to you. This will disengage your abdominal muscles and reduce the amount of pressure on the baby.

The position you choose in labor will help or hinder your process. By assuming upright positions you will help your baby enter the pelvis and apply more pressure on the cervix to help it dilate. Once you begin pushing, this upright position will allow you to use gravity to help you push as your body is aligned properly.

Once your cervix is fully dilated, you will begin to have the urge to push or bear down. It is during this portion of labor, known as the second stage of labor, that you will push your baby out. When you actively begin pushing, you will use your abdominals and your breathing, which is deeply related to your abdominal muscles, to help urge your baby into the world.

CHAPTER 14

Legs and Glutes

Your legs and glutes are very important parts of your body. You use them on a daily basis to stand, walk, lift, and bend. Strong legs and glutes also give you an advantage when it is time to give birth. You will use them to position yourself comfortably for labor and then for birth. By increasing the strength and tone during pregnancy, you help make this part of labor much easier.

Muscles

Your legs and glutes are the largest muscle groups in your body. They help you walk, bend, lift your legs, stabilize your body, and promote your back health. It is important to know something about these muscles as you exercise them. Being able to visualize where they are and how they work will make your workouts more effective.

Hip Flexors and Quadriceps

The hip flexors assist you in lifting your legs to the front. You use these muscles while walking up stairs or standing up on a step. They are located opposite of your glutes. If you sit a lot during the day, they may be shorter than normal. Exercise and stretching can help strengthen them so that they are more useful.

Your quadriceps are located in the front of your thighs. As you can see by the prefix *quad*, there are four main muscles in this group:

- Rectus femoris (the largest)
- Vastus medialis
- Vastus lateralis
- Vastus intermedius

The main function of this muscle group is to allow you to extend your leg from the knee, as in walking or bending.

Glutes (Buttocks)

Your buttocks are often referred to as your "glutes." This is actually a group of three muscles: gluteus maximus (the largest), gluteus medius, and gluteus minimus (smallest).

The more strengthened a muscle is, the more calories it burns at rest. So even if you are sleeping, muscle mass will be burning calories. Fatty tissue does not do this, even while you exercise. So the more muscles you have, the more calories you burn at rest.

The gluteus maximus helps you walk and jump. The gluteus medius helps with more lateral movement. The gluteus minimus is used to help rotate the leg outward. It is also located underneath the area where, one might say, you have saddlebags.

Thighs and Hamstrings

A special word needs to be said about your thighs, particularly your inner thighs. This area is one of the least worked areas of the body. And yet, it is also the one that will be called upon repeatedly in labor.

The inner thigh is called your hip adductor. It helps move your legs across the body, for example, in crossing your feet over each other, or doing dance steps. It also helps stabilize your knees. The outer thigh is called your hip abductor. This muscle helps move your foot away from your body and helps in stabilizing your hips and knees.

QUESTION

How can I prevent leg cramps at night?
Many pregnant women suffer from leg cramps, particularly at night. Well-toned and strengthened muscles will be less susceptible to this problem, which can be very painful. Stretching the lower leg just before bed and ensuring that you have plenty of calcium and potassium in your diet are ways to help alleviate this problem. Dehydration can also cause cramping, so drinking lots of fluids can also help prevent cramps.

The easiest way to remember the difference in their functions is to look at the prefix. To add to the body is to be a hip adductor—you are moving that leg inward, toward your body. The abductor moves away from the body.

The hamstrings are located in the back of your thighs. They function to bring your heel toward your glutes and to help you bend your knees. They do work with the other muscles in this area to produce a movement, such as bringing your leg up behind you. Many women find this area to be a tight area, which can cause pain. Stretching and warming up before a workout can help alleviate this problem.

Lower Leg

The calf muscles are located in the back of your leg, below the knee. The soleus and gastrocnemius muscles make up this muscle group. The soleus muscle lies underneath the gastrocnemius muscle, which is what you see when you look at your calf. These muscles help you stabilize the ankle joint and move when you lift your heel.

Your anterior tibialis, or shin muscle, is on the front part of your lower leg, under your knee. Unless you are suffering from shin splints, you probably don't pay much attention to this muscle, which is contracted as you lift the ball of your foot.

The Role of Glutes in Pregnancy

It might sound strange, but pregnancy is the perfect time to tone your legs and butt. It can help you identify different muscle groups and potential problem areas. It also gives you an advantage in labor as you prepare your body for the hard work of giving birth.

You do need to realize that your gluteal area is an area that is designed to accumulate fat deposits during pregnancy. This is your body's way of protecting you and your baby after birth should you need the extra fuel for feeding your baby. Breastfeeding and exercise are the best ways to remove this added fat on your body. So don't be concerned as your pregnancy progresses if you notice fat deposits being laid down in this area. It is not a sign that your workout efforts are failing. It is a sign that your body is doing an excellent job of preparing for your new baby.

Legs and Labor

When you think of labor, you probably have a television version in your mind. You might envision contractions and bed rest, coupled with funny breathing and screaming nasty things at those around you. Labor is much more than what you're shown on television. It's a combination of physical, mental, and emotional work.

During labor, it's clear that your uterus and abdominal muscles are working. What most pregnant women do not realize, however, is that their legs do a lot of work as well. We have learned about different positions that can be used to help facilitate an easier labor. Many of these positions require strong leg muscles to help support your body.

The Role Legs Play

During labor, your legs will carry you as you walk around to facilitate labor's progress. Your legs will help you assume positions to encourage your baby's descent into the birth canal. They will rock you in a chair and carry you to the shower or bathtub.

You will actually use your legs to assist you in pushing. While you won't actively push with your legs, you will have to hold them in different positions and use their force to assist you. Having strong muscles that are stretched and ready to go will be most beneficial. Using the muscles during pregnancy and actively preparing them for birth will give you the added benefit of stamina during labor.

FACT

Squatting, which really requires practice and leg strength, opens your pelvic outlet by an additional 10 percent. This position facilitates the birth of your baby and is often jokingly called the midwives' forceps. Practicing this position during pregnancy will help you to use it more effectively during birth. It also helps prevent the need for episiotomy and/or tearing of the perineum.

While you are in labor and you come to the second stage, or pushing phase of labor, you can also enlist the help of others around you in holding your legs in certain positions. While you can't get a lot of leg support while squatting, your partner, doula, or nurses can help hold up your body. They can also help hold your legs, particularly if you are very tired or have had epidural anesthesia.

Basically, any fitness program you do should include leg work. Both your legs and glutes will play an important part in your labor and recovery. They will also help you recover more quickly once your baby is born.

Leg Exercises for Strength and Tone

The good news about working out your lower extremities during pregnancy is that there are very few contraindications to these exercises. The majority are simple to do and can be done nearly anywhere, at any time. There are very few modifications needed because of your pregnancy.

Since these areas make up a large portion of your muscle mass, remember that they need attention, too. Everyday exercises (for example, walking) do help this area, but you need to make a concerted effort to strengthen the legs and glutes.

Lunge

Stand tall with feet shoulder-width apart and hands on hips or placed on the back of a chair or against a wall for added support. Maintain the proper posture of a straight back and gaze forward, while stepping two to three feet forward with your left foot. Your upper body should remain facing forward and straight. Be sure to keep your left knee from creeping past your toes, and keep in mind that leaning or twisting could cause injury. Lower your body until your left thigh is nearly parallel to the floor, again, keeping your knee behind your toes. Raise your body and bring your left foot back to starting position by pushing off of your left foot. Do eight to ten repetitions of this exercise and then repeat on the opposite side.

Reverse Lunge

Stand tall with feet shoulder-width apart and hands on hips or resting on the back of a chair or placed against a wall for added support. Maintain the proper posture of a straight back and gaze forward, while stepping two to three feet backward with your left leg. Your upper body should remain facing forward and straight. Be sure to keep your right knee from creeping past your toes, and keep in mind that leaning or twisting could cause injury. Lower your body until your right thigh is nearly parallel to the floor, again, keeping your knee behind your toes. Raise your body and bring your left foot back to starting position by pressing into your right foot. Do eight to ten repetitions of this exercise and then repeat on the opposite side.

Squat

This can help strengthen the muscles of your thighs to allow for an easier time at birth if you choose to give birth in this position. You can have assistance as you become familiar with the exercise by using a chair in front of you for extra support, keeping in mind that you should not lean forward on the chair. With your feet shoulder-width apart, slowly lower your body as if you were taking a seat in a chair behind you. Using your thighs and glutes, slowly lower yourself as far as you feel comfortable, without your knees creeping over your toes. Tighten your thighs and glutes and visualize their action as you use them to lift yourself back to the starting position. You will probably require some practice doing this exercise until you can do it alone and go down into a near-sitting position. Do ten squats, holding each one for five to ten seconds. Avoid bouncing in between squats.

ALERT

Varicose veins in the leg are not uncommon in pregnancy. If you find yourself with distended veins, be sure to show them to your doctor or midwife. You may need to wear support hose to help alleviate the problem. Elevating your feet above your heart also helps improve circulation. Watch for hot or painful spots, as it may indicate a blood clot. Let your practitioner know about this symptom right away.

Supported Squat (Wall Squat) with the Ball

Standing up straight with your back facing a wall, place the birth ball between you and the wall around the center of your back and press it into the wall using your back. Slowly walk your feet forward, leaning back into the ball for support. As you walk forward, the ball will roll up to the center of your back, between your shoulder blades. This allows you to do a squat without having to worry about being steady or having a partner. When you are lowered to the point where your thighs are parallel to the floor (keeping knees behind the toes), hold the pose for up to ten seconds, then slowly walk your feet back to their starting position, allowing the ball to roll back to the center of your lower back.

Calf Raises

If you feel you need support, you can perform this exercise facing the wall with palms on the wall at shoulder height. Slowly lift your feet, raising your heels, like standing on the tip of your toes, and slowly return to starting position. Do this eight to ten times and repeat with the other foot.

Exercises for Those Who Sit

If you find yourself sitting at a desk all day, you may not feel like you're getting your legs stretched and exercised. You might even suffer from pain or swelling in the legs. To minimize the pain and swelling associated with pregnancy, be sure to drink plenty of water, stretch your legs often, and do focus at least some of your fitness time on your legs.

Leg Extensions

Sit on the edge of a chair. Use a dumbbell as a weight. Place it between your feet. Hold on to the edges of the chair and begin to raise your legs slowly, bringing the dumbbell with you. This will strengthen and flex your quads and glutes. Slowly return to your starting position. Repeat this exercise ten times. Be careful not to use too great a weight or to go too quickly.

During the workday you may want to walk around a bit more to ensure good circulation. Rather than letting work pile up before you distribute it, consider making several trips as the work comes across your desk. Sure, you might walk to the copier two or three times more than you might before, but it will help your legs and body feel better during the day. Take the stairs when appropriate and walk around your neighborhood. Do whatever it takes to keep your legs moving!

Thigh Abduction

While seated in a chair, place a small ball between your thighs. Keeping your back straight, squeeze your thighs together until your knees are touching, and hold for five seconds. Release and return to starting position. Repeat ten times for one set. Perform three sets throughout the day.

Tush Tightener

While sitting in a chair with your back straight, squeeze your butt muscles until you feel your body slightly lift from your chair. Hold the squeeze for five to ten seconds, and release for one repetition. Do ten repetitions for one set, and aim for three sets daily.

Stretches

With stretches that focus on your legs, butt, and calves, you can help your body release tension from the newly challenging movements that result from gradual pregnancy weight gain. If you find yourself feeling tight or swollen, you can take a few minutes to perform a couple of quick stretches that will help loosen muscles and relieve tension.

Pelvic Rock/Pelvic Tilt

This is the perfect exercise for backaches in pregnancy. It will not only help prevent them, but cure them as well. Assume an all-fours position, on your hands and knees. Think of holding your back in its natural alignment. Then tuck only your pelvis in, bringing your pubic bone toward your neck. Be sure to move only your pelvis. If it helps, have someone hold your pelvis so that you can learn to isolate this area. Later, this exercise can be done in different positions. You need to do two sets of twenty repetitions of the pelvic tilts.

Side Lying Stretches

Lying on your right side, stretch your left arm over your body as if reaching for something above your head. Focus on extending the arm as well as the leg and body. This should feel like a good tension release. Hold this pose for about ten seconds. Repeat on the left side.

Limitations and Modifications

Because the muscles of your legs and butt are the largest in the body, the lactic acid that can build up as a result of exercise can cause excruciating stiffness and tightness. In order to prevent pain and injury as a result from lower-body workouts, it is absolutely imperative that you warm up your legs prior to your workout and stretch following every workout.

ESSENTIAL

The pelvic rock or tilt can become your best pregnancy exercise to prepare you for labor and delivery. You can learn to do it standing up, or while leaning against a wall for added comfort. In fact, if you take a canister of unopened tennis balls and place it behind the small of your back prior to doing the pelvic rocks, you can manage to give yourself a quick massage.

The muscles of your leg and butt only really benefit from exercises performed with two to three days between workouts. Again, being the largest muscle group in the body, your lower half will need ample time to rest and recover before it can be expected to perform another bout of exercises at full potential. By allowing two full days between leg and butt workouts, you can focus your efforts on arms, abs, chest, and back, and max out the benefits from all body parts . . . without unnecessary discomfort.

Exercising your legs and bottom is very important. It can be so easy to focus on other areas during pregnancy. The benefits you will get from the exercise you do now will follow you to birth. This will also help make weight loss easier once your baby has been born.

CHAPTER 15

First Trimester

The first trimester of pregnancy is a whirlwind of excitement, newness, and responsibility. The first trimester is the first part of your life caring for the child you carry, and how you care for yourself in these first couple of months will directly affect the health and development of your baby. Newly pregnant, you may be having some new pregnancy symptoms, or you may be one of the lucky ones who has none. Either way, your focus in the first trimester should be on your diet, exercise, and quality of life.

In Case You Didn't Know . . .

Your first trimester of pregnancy ends at about twelve weeks, or three months after your last menstrual period. Your doctor may discuss your progress in weeks, which are measured from the first day of your last menstrual period—the day your doctor uses to calculate your due date and the baby's gestational age. Since it is usually impossible to pinpoint the exact date of ovulation and the date of conception, medical experts use your last menstrual period as the starting point for your next nine months. Basically, this means that the first week of your pregnancy is actually the week that you started your last period.

In terms of your lifestyle, it is important to take note that everything you eat, drink, and do will directly affect your baby. Experts don't exactly understand how the mother and baby divvy up the nutrients, but we do know that the baby lives on the nutrients from the mother's diet and the nutrients already stored in her bones and tissues. The baby's health and proper growth are directly related to the mother's diet before and during pregnancy. It is essential for both you and your baby that you make sure you are eating a healthy diet. You should also be taking a prenatal vitamin at this time to ensure you are getting all of the nutrients that are essential to a healthy pregnancy, including folic acid, calcium, and iron. Good nutrition and a healthy lifestyle are essential throughout your entire pregnancy, though certain nutritional considerations may be more important at different stages along the way. In your first trimester, important nutritional considerations include folic acid intake, prevention of malnutrition, and dehydration.

What's Going On

Along with changes in your baby's development, you will experience changes in your own body. The embryo secretes a hormone called human chorionic gonadotropin (hCG), or the pregnancy hormone. This hormone triggers your first signs of pregnancy. In your first trimester, you may begin to experience nausea, vomiting, dizziness, headaches, a feeling of fullness or bloating, light cramping, constipation, poor appetite, frequent urination, and breast tenderness. You may need to go to the bathroom more often. This is because your growing uterus is pressing on your bladder and because hormones may be affecting your body's fluid balance.

Around week eight, your uterus grows from the size of your fist to about the size of a grapefruit, which can cause some mild cramping or pain in your lower abdomen or sides. Some of these problems will decrease as you continue with your pregnancy.

Moodiness and anxiety can surface and make you feel like you are on an emotional roller coaster. Feeling happy one day and crabby the next is completely normal, due partly to fluctuating and very high levels of hormones. For many women, this moodiness and anxiety continues throughout pregnancy. You may begin to notice changes in your figure by the end of your first trimester. Your breasts have become larger, and you may notice that your waistline is beginning to expand just a bit.

ALERT

Weight gain in the first trimester should be about 2 to 4 pounds. Keep in mind that excessive weight gain during pregnancy can be a problem for both you and your baby. A normal weight gain during pregnancy, for women who begin at a normal weight, is 25 to 35 pounds. If your weight gain during the first trimester seems abnormal, speak with your doctor.

Worried about Lack of Appetite?

During the first trimester, a lack of appetite can be very normal. It is normal to experience nausea or morning sickness and to have a constant feeling of fullness that may cause you to eat less or just not want to eat. Don't make yourself too crazy about your lack of appetite—your good nutritional stores are nourishing the baby at this time. Even though you shouldn't worry too much, you should still do all you can to eat as nutritiously as possible. Try eating small meals throughout the day, eating starchy foods before getting out of bed, and staying away from foods with strong odors. Do the best you can to keep up your nutritional intake during this time, and keep in mind that by your second trimester these feelings should diminish.

Food Aversions

Food aversions during pregnancy are almost as common as food cravings. It is quite normal in pregnancy to suddenly be disgusted by the taste, sight, and/or smell of a certain food or beverage that you have always enjoyed. Food aversions can go as quickly, and they come and differ from woman to woman as much as cravings do. Meat is probably the most common food aversion, though other popular aversions include water, coffee, tea, fried and fatty foods, highly spiced foods, alcohol, and eggs.

Like food cravings, the cause of food aversions is pretty much unknown. There is some evidence that hormonal changes in pregnant women cause a heightened sense of smell, which may impact foods that are craved or avoided. Some speculate that food aversions are your body's way of telling you that you should avoid certain foods or beverages that are not good for you during pregnancy. Developing an aversion to coffee or alcohol can help you avoid something you shouldn't be having anyway.

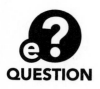

QUESTION

Is it unhealthy to have an aversion to vegetables during my first trimester?
It is common for women to have food aversions even to healthy foods such as vegetables. Try drinking vegetable juice instead of eating whole vegetables. You can also eat more fruit, since many of them contain some of the same nutrients as vegetables. Keep taking your prenatal vitamins to ensure you are getting all of the nutrients that your body needs at this time. If you have a temporary aversion to a healthy food, make substitutions. If you're not sure what to substitute, be sure to speak to a dietitian.

On the other hand, some experts worry about aversions to foods that you should be eating and that can cause nutritional deficiencies. If you develop an aversion to specific healthy foods such as milk, make sure you try substituting something nutritionally similar such as yogurt. If you develop an aversion to water, it is essential that you do something to replace it. Try drinking water flavored with 100-percent fruit juice. Remember that food aversions come and go quickly. If you can't stand the sight of a food one day, make sure you try it again soon.

Fighting the Fatigue

Pregnancy, especially during the first trimester, can work your body overtime. It is normal to feel a little worn out when you are busy building another person! You may feel tired to the point of complete exhaustion. In addition to the obvious reasons for being tired, vomiting and lack of appetite can also zap your energy, as well as rob you of some essential nutrients. Hormonal changes in particular can cause fatigue. Being worried and anxious about being pregnant, along with frequent trips to the bathroom at night, can rob you of needed sleep. Most of these problems diminish in the second trimester, and you will feel much more alert. Feelings of fatigue usually surface again around the seventh month, when you are carrying more weight around.

You can't always completely fight fatigue, but you can give it a valiant try. Here are a few tips you can follow to help yourself deal with fatigue:

- Go to bed early and at a regular time to keep your body on a regular schedule. Shoot for at least nine to ten hours of sleep a night if your schedule allows it.
- Take short fifteen-minute catnaps during the day. Be careful of sleeping too much and interfering with your sleep at night. Your body will tell you when you need to rest.
- Keep as active as you can during the day with regular exercise. Even though you may feel too tired to even think about exercise, just a short walk during the day can help energize you.
- Take short breaks throughout the day to do some stretching and breathing exercises.
- Eat small, frequent meals throughout the day, and make sure you are eating a healthy diet that includes all the food groups. Eating throughout the day will fuel and help energize your body all day long.
- Stay hydrated by drinking plenty of water throughout the day, and make sure to cut back on your caffeine intake.

- Eat energy-boosting foods, especially in the middle of the day. Include a good source of protein as well as carbohydrates, such as peanut butter on bread, grilled chicken and veggies on pita bread, chicken noodle soup, grilled cheese sandwich, or an egg white with cheese on a whole-wheat bagel.
- Good, energy-boosting snacks to nibble on during the day include dried fruit, fortified cereal and milk, yogurt with fruit and granola, cheese and crackers, nuts and/or seeds, frozen grapes or bananas, a granola bar, a milkshake, or vegetable juice.
- Don't be afraid to ask for help with household chores that may be zapping your energy, and do as many of your chores as you can while seated.
- Stay within your weight-gain guidelines. The more weight you have to carry around, the more fatigued you will feel.
- Ensure you are taking your prenatal vitamins, as directed by your doctor.
- If your exhaustion becomes debilitating or continues into your second trimester, speak with your doctor. Extreme exhaustion can be a sign of other problems such as anemia or thyroid problems.

What's Happening with Baby?

Even though this is just the beginning, and your baby is tinier than you can probably imagine, it's a very big time for both of you! The development that occurs in these first few weeks is so rapid, and yet so essential to the healthy natural progression that will bring your baby from the bundle of cells he starts out as to the bundle of joy you'll soon deliver. You may feel pregnant, but you may not. You may start to show, but you may not. Regardless of what's happening on the outside, the miracles taking place in your body, each and every day, are nothing short of remarkable.

Your First Month (1 to 4 Weeks)

About two weeks after the first day of your last menstrual period, your ovary released an egg into the fallopian tube. Your actual pregnancy began when that egg was fertilized by a sperm cell.

Over the next week, the fertilized egg grows into a group of cells called a blastocyst. Once the blastocyst completes its journey down the fallopian tube, it implants in the uterus and divides into two parts. One half of the blastocyst attaches to the wall of the uterus and becomes the placenta while the other half develops into the embryo. This group of cells is already composed of different layers. The outer layer eventually becomes the nervous system, skin, and hair. The middle layer becomes bones, cartilage, muscles, circulatory system, kidneys, and sex organs. The inner layer becomes the respiratory and digestive organs.

The implantation of the egg into the uterus triggers the beginning of hormonal and physical changes. The amniotic sac, which cushions the fetus in the months ahead, begins to form. The early stages of the placenta and umbilical cord are visible and under rapid construction.

During the first month of pregnancy, the embryo looks like a tadpole. The neural tube, which will become the brain and spinal cord, starts to come together. A very primitive face begins to form, with large dark circles where the eyes will be. The mouth, lower jaw, and throat also begin to develop. The baby's blood cells are taking shape, and circulation will soon begin. By the end of the first month, the embryo is about a quarter of an inch long and is smaller than a grain of rice.

FACT

The placenta is the interface that provides all the nutrients the baby needs, including oxygen, and takes care of waste disposal. It also produces the hormones progesterone and estriol, which are produced to help maintain a healthy pregnancy. The placenta develops in the uterus just twelve days after conception.

Your Second Month (5 to 8 Weeks)

You may not look pregnant yet, but by the second month of your pregnancy, plenty is going on. Major body organs are beginning to develop, including the heart, brain, kidneys, liver, intestines, appendix, lungs, and body systems. The baby's facial features continue to develop. The baby's ears, fingers, toes, and eyes begin to form. Tiny buds that will become the baby's arms and legs are forming. The digestive tract and sensory organs are now beginning to develop.

During this time, bone starts to replace cartilage. The baby's heart starts its contractions, which will become distinct heartbeats within the next week. The eyelids form and grow—though sealed shut—and nostrils begin to form.

The neural tube will eventually connect the brain and spinal cord, and by about the fifth week it closes. Blood circulation becomes evident at this time. The placenta and amniotic sac continue to develop. By the end of the second month, the embryo has started to look more like a person than a tadpole. It measures about 1 inch long and weighs less than ⅓ ounce.

Your Third Month (9 to 12 Weeks)

During your third month of pregnancy, the embryo has developed into a fetus. The baby is active, even though you may not yet be able to feel the activity. All major organs, muscles, and nerves are formed. The mouth has twenty buds that will eventually become teeth. The irises of the eyes are now forming. The liver, intestines, brain, and lungs are now beginning to function on their own. At around week eleven, it is possible to hear the "swooshing" sound of the baby's heartbeat for the first time with a special instrument called a Doppler sound-wave stethoscope.

ESSENTIAL

A Doppler stethoscope uses ultrasound to listen to the heartbeat of the fetus. The device is sometimes called a Doptone. The Doppler may be routinely used during your prenatal visits.

Several of the baby's ribs are now visible, and tissue that will eventually form bones is developing around the baby's head, arms, and legs. By the end of your first trimester, or third month, your baby is fully formed. Your little one has arms, hands, fingers, feet, and toes. Fingers and toes are separate, and they now have soft nails. Your baby's reproductive organs are developing, and the circulatory and urinary systems are working. The liver is producing bile.

Throughout the remainder of your pregnancy, the baby's body organs will mature and the fetus will gain weight, become longer, and fully develop. By the end of your third month, your baby is about four inches in length and weighs about 1 ounce. The most critical point of formation of the organs is finished, and your chance of miscarriage at this point drops considerably.

What Your Body Needs

The nutritional needs for pregnant women should be more focused on *quality* than *quantity*. Your diet should include an additional 150–300 calories, which is the equivalent of an additional salad or extra helping of rice. Rather than focusing on the extra food you could or should be eating, try to consider the nutrition of foods you include in your diet . . . maximizing the nutrients that can help promote the healthy growth of you and your baby. Plus, if you happen to experience one of the less-than-desirable pregnancy symptoms like nausea or food aversions, you'll want to pack as much nutrition into the foods you are able to eat and keep down.

ALERT

Malnutrition is defined as a state of impaired health caused by inadequate intake or inadequate digestion of nutrients. It can be caused by not eating a balanced diet, not eating enough, digestive problems, absorption problems, or other medical conditions.

Here are just a few ideas that can help you ensure you're making the best diet decisions that will benefit you and your baby throughout your pregnancy . . . and beyond!

- **Eat the Rainbow:** Try to include as many colors in your diet as possible. From vibrant reds, yellows, and blues to deep oranges and greens, it is absolutely essential that you consume foods packed with nutrients in order to optimize the quality of your health and the health of your baby.

- **Snack More:** Especially in the first trimester, it can be difficult to find the perfect amount of food that will satisfy your hunger, but not make you nauseous. If you find yourself feeling queasy or over-full faster than usual, eating smaller snack-size meals more often can help you avoid discomfort following your mealtimes.
- **Variety Is Key:** Even if you feel like crackers are the only food you can eat without visiting the bathroom afterward, try foods that offer up more nutrition from other food groups. Sometimes, texture can be more of a nausea trigger than taste, so if you find yourself avoiding foods of a certain consistency, try including those same foods prepared in a different way, or foods of the same food group that have a different texture altogether.
- **Get Creative:** If you're finding it difficult to sit down and consume an entire meal or snack, opt for a smoothie instead. You can combine fruits, vegetables, yogurts, or teas together in different combinations without losing any of the nutrients you need.

The first trimester is a very important time for both mom and baby in terms of growth, development, and growing accustomed to a new way of life. Whether you're trying to clean up your diet or have one at all, it is crucial to pack the right nutrition into every bite. Forego the junk food, sugary snacks, and sodas, and opt for the naturally nutritious foods your body (and your baby) deserve.

Preventing Dehydration

You need extra fluids in pregnancy for your increased blood volume and for amniotic fluid. Keeping properly hydrated can also help prevent urinary tract infections, constipation, and hemorrhoids, all common problems during pregnancy. Dehydration can be a concern in the first trimester if you are experiencing vomiting. Vomiting can remove vital fluids that your body needs to keep you in balance. Dehydration may also be a concern if you are not eating the proper amount of calories and if you are not drinking fluids due to feelings of nausea or fullness. If your doctor is concerned about dehydration, he may use a urine test to determine if you are maintaining a proper fluid level.

You should aim to drink at least eight to ten glasses of fluids per day. If you are nauseated, fluids such as ginger ale or lemon tea can help soothe your stomach and contribute to your fluid intake. If you are vomiting, products such as Gatorade can help to replenish electrolytes. Some women who have a hard time getting plain water down do well with lemonade and/or juice. Stay away from caffeinated beverages—caffeine can act as a diuretic and compound the problem of dehydration. If you feel signs of dehydration, such as dry lips or a dry mouth, make sure you are drinking enough fluids. Be careful not to fill up on too many fluids at meals and not leave room for food. Drink your fluids between meals instead of with your meals.

ALERT

It is not unusual to be thirstier during pregnancy. However, being excessively thirsty can be a sign of other medical conditions, such as diabetes. If severe thirst is forcing you to drink large amounts of fluids, tell your doctor immediately.

Exercising: Baby on Board!

Some women choose to wait until the end of their first trimester to begin exercising, though there is no real reason to do so if you are only experiencing normal first-trimester symptoms. In fact, there are many references out there that point to exercise as a way to relieve some of the problems like nausea, fatigue, and dietary concerns. The key to the appropriate amount of exercise in the first trimester, particularly for those who have not exercised before, is to avoid overdoing it. Remember to let your body be your guide.

Start with easy exercises for beginners, like simple exercise routines. Walking or swimming, for example, can be continued throughout pregnancy and offer numerous benefits. Even bicycling, stationary or regular, can be continued for much of pregnancy. Try creating your own routine that fulfills your needs for exercise while enhancing your body's ability to gestate.

Exercise for the First Trimester

During the beginning part of pregnancy there are very few exercises that you need to avoid. Because your uterus is not very big, you don't yet have some of the special concerns that you will have in later parts of pregnancy, and you still have a lot of mobility.

The main point to focus on is *how* you are exercising. Practicing good posture will help keep you and your baby safe while allowing you a good workout. Be sure to watch for signs of problems while exercising, particularly dehydration. Make sure you drink plenty of water before, during, and after exercising.

Keeping an eye on the signs and signals your body is sending you during this pregnancy will help you avoid certain problems. By listening, you and your practitioner can learn to tell when changes are going on that may indicate early labor, poor fetal growth, and other complications, although complications are not always predictable in pregnancy. If you experienced these problems in a previous pregnancy, you might be at a higher risk for a repeated scenario.

Other than these few simple precautions, your exercise limitations in the first trimester will be the same ones you would normally have. Anything that your body responds negatively to while you exercise is also contraindicated.

How much or how often you exercise during your pregnancy will largely be determined by your pregnancy history, as well as other factors such as your current fitness level. If you have had problems with preterm labor or other difficulties in a previous pregnancy, it is very important to discuss this with your doctor or midwife. While this may not affect your current pregnancy at all, more monitoring is generally indicated.

CHAPTER 16

Second Trimester

You're officially in your second trimester! You've weathered the ups and downs of the first trimester, and you've made it to the part of pregnancy most moms refer to as "the easy period"! With your baby bump proudly advertising your mom-to-be status, and a refreshed feeling that comes with the subsided symptoms of your first trimester, you can be free to enjoy pregnancy for all it can be. Continue traveling the path to best health, and you ensure that same quality of health for your baby, too.

In Case You Didn't Know . . .

In your second trimester of pregnancy, you will begin to gain more of your pregnancy weight. You should experience a steady weight gain of about 1 pound per week in your second trimester, although the rate of weight gain differs from woman to woman. Even though you may be losing your girlish figure, keep in mind that proper weight gain is a good thing in pregnancy. No matter how much some pregnant women hate to admit it, they struggle with their changing figures. Don't beat yourself up about feeling a little unhappy. It is very normal, and you should give yourself permission to experience both the joys and frustrations of watching your body change in so many ways.

Stay Positive

With your doctor's permission, develop a regular exercise program and stick to it. Women who exercise regularly during pregnancy maintain a higher self-esteem. Remaining active throughout your pregnancy can help lessen feelings of depression, stress, and worries over weight gain and body image. Define the attributes you find attractive in yourself and accentuate them to help make you feel better about yourself. Pamper yourself by doing things that make you feel good and that will help you to build your self-image. Keeping your weight gain within healthy, recommended limits can help make you feel better about your body size. Too much or too little weight gain can sabotage your efforts for a positive body and self-image. Most important, keep your eye on the prize at the end of the journey. Each time your self-image seems to slip, think about that beautiful, healthy baby you are going to have. Keep in mind that this change is temporary. There will be plenty of time to regain your figure after your baby is born. Take a positive attitude and see the beauty and importance of the changes in your body. It is up to you!

What's Going On

The changes in the second trimester can be quite dramatic. You might wake up one morning and feel like a cloud has been lifted. You may not even feel very pregnant in the classic sense of nausea and grouchiness. Where you may have felt exhausted, cranky, mentally foggy, and an overall sense of being uncomfortable, the second trimester will probably be your turn-around point where you get to feel like yourself again. Not only will you be feeling better accustomed to being pregnant, but you may get the sense that your body is, too.

If you weren't showing much in your first trimester and felt like wearing a sign that read, "I'm pregnant!" to let people in on your excitement, your second trimester will take care of your hidden condition by being the time when you "pop" your baby belly that will let everyone know you're expecting. With your expanding belly, you get to explore the whole new world of ever more stylish maternity wear that will help you feel comfortable *and* stylish. With more energy, less discomfort, a new wardrobe, and a proud baby bump, what's not to feel great about? Add to all of the second-trimester greatness the fact that you get to feel your baby move for the first time, and you may just feel like it can't get any better!

Be sure to take advantage of this pregnancy period. Use the time to get out and enjoy life. Take more walks; spend more time doing things you enjoy. Simply enjoy the pregnancy.

Those Crazy Cravings!

Though there is no agreed-upon explanation for them, food cravings are extremely common during pregnancy. There will be foods you can't seem to stomach, and there will be foods you just can't get enough of. Some experts blame raging hormones. Just as some women crave certain foods during their menstrual cycle due to hormones, the same thing happens during pregnancy. Some believe that in an opposite case from food aversions, the body's craving of a certain food signals a need for some nutrient or nutrients. Alternately, some scientists believe that cravings are the way the body takes care of getting its extra calories. Some of the most commonly craved foods for pregnant women include citrus fruits, chips, dairy products, spicy foods, ice cream, chocolate, and other sweet foods. In fact, women tend to crave sweet foods more during their second trimester than at any other time in their pregnancy. One thing is undeniable: A woman's taste preferences do change throughout her pregnancy.

Should You Give In?

Your food cravings may not necessarily be a problem or cause imbalances in your diet if you seem to be craving healthier foods, like fruit or milk. But what do you do when you are craving that hot fudge sundae? If high-calorie, high-sugar, and/or high-fat foods are what you crave, you will have to exercise mind over matter on occasion. Giving in to cravings every time, especially if they are frequent and you are craving high-calorie foods, is a good way to pack on more pounds than you intended. In addition, if you seem to be craving and eating a lot of one certain food and not eating much of anything else, you may become deficient in important nutrients over time.

Do your best to fit your cravings into a nutritionally balanced diet. As long as you are eating a balanced diet and getting the essential nutrients you need for you and your baby, giving in to your cravings once in a while is probably fine. The bottom line is that indulging in your food cravings in moderation is harmless. You may find that your food cravings get less intense as you progress through your pregnancy.

Helpful Hints

Try some of these helpful hints to work cravings into your balanced diet:

- Eat a good, healthy breakfast. Skipping meals such as breakfast can increase the cravings for certain foods later in the day.
- Eat plenty of complex carbohydrates, such as whole-wheat breads, brown rice, whole-grain cereals, and pasta. Complex carbohydrates take longer to digest and therefore help to keep blood sugar levels consistent. Dips in blood sugar can cause cravings.
- Work the foods you crave into a nutritional diet. If you crave chocolate, try chocolate milk. If you crave ice cream, add sliced fruit such as bananas or strawberries to your ice cream to give it a nutritional punch.
- Take a closer look at your total diet. Keep a food diary for a week or so and review it to make sure you are eating a balanced diet and getting the nutrients that you need.
- Indulge in your healthy cravings and try to find healthier alternatives to your unhealthy ones most of the time. For example, substitute non-fat frozen yogurt if you crave ice cream, or pretzels if you crave chips.

- Think small when it comes to the portion sizes of your higher-calorie cravings. If you crave chocolate candy, instead of a whole candy bar, grab a one-bite serving.
- Stay active and exercise regularly. Exercise can help curb hunger and tame cravings.
- Make sure you have the emotional support that you need. Pregnancy can put you on a mood-altering roller coaster, and these mood swings may cause you to turn to food for comfort.
- If you crave nonfood substances and cannot resist the craving, talk to your doctor.

ALERT

The craving for nonfood items (for example, dirt, chalk, toothpaste, clay, soap, or laundry starch) when pregnant is actually a disorder known as pica. Eating nonfood items is not safe as they may interfere with nutrient absorption or may be toxic or contain parasites. You should contact your doctor immediately if you experience frequent cravings for nonfood items.

Healthier Alternatives

There are always healthier alternatives that you can turn to when you crave certain foods. It's fine to indulge on occasion, but try healthier alternatives more often. Keep in mind, though, that even healthier alternatives in large amounts can add unwanted calories and pounds.

Instead Of	Try
Potato chips	Pretzels, unbuttered popcorn, or baked tortilla chips
Ice cream	Fruit smoothies, flavored kefir, nonfat yogurt or frozen yogurt, sorbet, frozen juice bar, or sherbet
Colas	Fruit juice or water flavored with a little fruit juice
Doughnuts	Whole-wheat bagel with low-fat cream cheese and/or jelly
Cake	Angel-food cake topped with fresh fruit
Apple pie	Applesauce with cinnamon
Cookies	Plain or cinnamon-coated graham crackers, vanilla wafers, gingersnaps, or animal cookies

Instead Of	Try
Chocolate bar	Fat-free chocolate milk or hot chocolate
Cupcake	Reduced fat or fat-free muffin
Sour cream	Low-fat sour cream or plain nonfat yogurt
Cheesecake	Low-fat pudding or flavored low-fat yogurt
Sweets	Raisins or other dried fruit, fruited gelatin, flavored rice cakes

What's Happening with Baby?

By your second trimester, your baby is well developed. This stage of the pregnancy can be very exciting because you may start to feel your baby move at about eighteen to twenty-two weeks. If this is not your first pregnancy, you may even be able to feel movement earlier, at sixteen to eighteen weeks. Your baby looks like a small person now and is continuing to develop every week during this period.

Your Fourth Month (13 to 16 Weeks)

By your fourth month of pregnancy, your baby's fingers and toes are well defined. Eyelids, eyebrows, and nails are formed. Hair is starting to grow on top of the baby's head, and facial features are more prominent. The teeth and bones are becoming harder. The baby is moving her arms and legs and can even suck her thumb, yawn, and stretch. The baby is starting to now respond to outside stimuli. The nervous system is beginning to function, and the reproductive organs and genitalia are now fully developed. At this point your doctor may be able tell through an ultrasound if you are having a boy or a girl. The baby's heartbeat is now undeniably audible through an instrument called a Doppler. By the end of your fourth month, the baby is about six inches long and weighs somewhere around 4 ounces.

Your Fifth Month (17 to 20 Weeks)

During your fifth month of pregnancy, hair on the head, eyebrows, and eyelashes are filling in. A soft, fine hair, called lanugo, covers the baby's body. Meant to protect the baby, lanugo is usually shed by the end of the baby's first week of life. Fat is beginning to form on the baby's body to help him stay warm and to aid in metabolism. The lungs, circulatory, and urinary systems are now in working condition. At this point, the retinas in the eyes are sensitive to light. The baby's skin is developing and appears transparent. Your baby can hear sounds such as your voice and heartbeat as well as sounds outside of your body. During this month, you may begin to feel the baby move as his muscles begin to develop. As the baby continues to develop, you will notice more movement. By the end of the fifth month, the baby is about ten inches long and weighs anywhere from 8 ounces to 1 pound.

FACT

At this point, you should start sleeping on your side because the circulation is best for mom and baby that way. By the time you get to your fourth or fifth month, lying on your stomach or your back can put extra pressure on your growing uterus and may decrease circulation to the baby.

Your Sixth Month (21 to 25 Weeks)

During your sixth month, the baby is continuing to gain fat to keep its body warm. His or her growth rate is slowing down, but bodily systems such as digestion are continuing to mature. Buds for the permanent teeth are beginning to form, and the baby's muscles are getting stronger. The baby is very active and will respond to sounds and movement. The baby's body is becoming better proportioned. It is beginning to produce white blood cells that will help the baby fight infection and disease. You may begin to tell when the baby has hiccups by the jerking motions you feel. The baby's skin is more opaque than transparent and is wrinkled as the baby grows into it. The heartbeat at this point can be heard more easily through a stethoscope, depending on the baby's position. By the end of the sixth month, your baby measures approximately twelve inches in length and somewhere around 2 pounds.

What Your Body Needs

As with your entire pregnancy, good nutrition and proper weight gain are essential during your second trimester. During this period, most women begin to experience decreased symptoms of morning sickness (though some may get morning sickness throughout pregnancy). It's a good thing these symptoms decrease for most because, starting now, you need to begin to boost your calorie intake. The nutritional concerns in this stage of pregnancy come from the digestive troubles that most women begin to experience.

As your pregnancy progresses into the second trimester, your baby continues to grow, which causes your stomach to work a little slower. Some women experience an intolerance to milk products at this time. Since calcium and other nutrients in dairy products are so essential to good health, especially during pregnancy, it is important to find an alternative. Other digestive problems women may experience as they enter the second trimester include gas, indigestion, and heartburn. Constipation can become a problem during the second trimester and continue until the end of your pregnancy. It is important to deal with these discomforts so that they don't interfere with your efforts to eat a healthy diet and don't turn into more complex complications.

Exercising: Belly on Board!

In your second trimester, you may be feeling the best you've felt all pregnancy! If your practitioner has cleared you for exercise during this pregnancy, and you've been working out since before you became pregnant or throughout this pregnancy, good for you! If you're just getting started in the fitness area for this pregnancy, good for you, too, because it's never too late to reap the benefits. Maintaining a feel-good exercise regimen in your second trimester can be easy and enjoyable, as long as you keep your body's new changes in mind, and remember a couple of guidelines that will keep you and your baby safe well into the third trimester.

Center of Gravity

During the second trimester, your center of gravity will begin to switch. It's something so subtle you are unlikely to detect much of anything. However, some women do report feeling a bit more clumsy at this point than before they became pregnant.

This is the time to give up high heels, walking on stilts, and anything else you might do that requires a lot of balance. For your exercise routines, this will mean you need to be constantly aware of your footing. Wear sensible shoes to avoid slipping and falling.

ALERT

Do not exercise in stocking feet, or even walk around the house in stocking feet if you can help it. Always use the handrails when you take the stairs. Use good body mechanics when getting up or down from sitting or lying positions. This is particularly true of places where falls are more likely, such as the pool or bathtub.

Lying on Your Back

It was a long-held belief that pregnant women should not lie on their backs after the sixteenth week of pregnancy. The theory behind this was that after this point in pregnancy, the uterus was so large that lying on your back decreased the blood flow from the vena cava (the main vein running down your posterior side) to the uterus and your baby, also lowering your blood pressure and affecting blood flow return from your legs.

FACT

Maternal supine hypotension syndrome can occur while sleeping on your back. The good news is that most of the time, you would wake up upon feeling these symptoms. Generally, you're not even aware of why you awoke; you just naturally change positions and go back to sleep.

This condition, called *maternal supine hypotension syndrome*, was never truly studied until recently. When the studies were done, it was found that many women didn't actually experience any of the symptoms of complications. This has led the medical world to believe that short periods of exercise on the back during the latter trimesters may be acceptable if you do not suffer from maternal supine hypotension syndrome.

Signs for maternal supine hypotension syndrome include:

- Dizziness
- Shortness of breath
- Passing out (extremely rare)

If you experience any of these while lying on your back, simply roll to your side until you feel you have recovered.

Keep in Mind . . .

Unlike your first trimester when nausea, vomiting, and fatigue reigned supreme, your second trimester is probably less exhausting. In fact, most women find this to be the best phase of pregnancy. Don't be concerned if you wouldn't quite put it that way. Remember, the range of "normal" varies widely.

ESSENTIAL

Even if you're feeling and looking great in this second part of pregnancy, there may be reasons to stop or modify your exercise routine. Generally, your doctor or midwife will discuss this need with you, but you should always feel comfortable bringing the subject up with him or her, or cutting back on your own.

Placenta Previa

As previously discussed, placenta previa is a condition in which the placenta covers all or part of the cervix. This actually comes in degrees from a full previa, where the entire cervix is covered by the placenta, to a marginal or partial previa, where only part of the cervix is covered. You might be diagnosed with a previa if you have bleeding or a mid-trimester ultrasound.

The good news is that over 95 percent of all placenta previas will naturally resolve themselves without you ever lifting a finger. The reason this happens is that the lower segment of the uterus does much of its growth in the latter half of the second trimester and in the third trimester. When this growth occurs, the placenta "moves" away from the cervix, resolving the problem.

If the placenta previa does not resolve itself by the end of pregnancy, a cesarean section is planned. A baby cannot be born through the placenta. If labor begins, bleeding may endanger you or the baby due to blood loss.

When it comes to exercise, your restrictions will largely depend on the extent of your previa and whether or not you've had any bleeding. If you have an appointment for an ultrasound and are told about the previa, discontinue all exercise until you talk to your doctor or midwife about the safety of resuming exercise.

Anemia

Anemia is also known as iron deficiency. Many pregnant women have this very common problem. It is most likely to be diagnosed in the second trimester of pregnancy because of routine blood work done at your practitioner's office. Your red blood cells act as your body's oxygen-carrying messengers in your blood. Pregnancy demands more oxygen because you need oxygen for your baby as well as for your normal needs. When you are anemic, this ability is decreased.

FACT

In this part of pregnancy, you will see a dramatic increase in your blood volume. If you have your blood tested for anemia at this juncture, you might be given a false diagnosis of anemia, because it takes the red blood cells a bit to catch up with their production. Never hesitate to ask to be retested.

Signs of anemia include:

- Fatigue
- Loss of energy
- Shortness of breath

- Weakness
- Paleness
- Low blood pressure

Even if your doctor or midwife doesn't test your blood for anemia, be sure to report these symptoms at your visits. While you may put it off as being just another part of pregnancy, anemia is something that can greatly affect you, even at the time of birth. You don't wish to take the risks associated with anemia when they can be easily treated, usually with just some minor dietary changes.

If you are anemic, you may need to back down on your exercise levels a bit. As you can see, the symptoms of anemia would make it difficult to exercise anyway. As you build your iron stores back up, and as your iron levels rise and become less affected by anemia, you can gradually increase your workouts.

Preterm Labor

As opposed to late miscarriage, which is technically defined by many states as either a specific gestation, or a specific fetal weight, no matter the condition of the baby at birth, preterm labor is defined as any labor or series of contractions that occur before thirty-seven weeks' gestation (from your last menstrual period). The risk of preterm labor is that if your baby is born before it is ready, it can suffer severe health consequences, including many that are life-threatening. Your doctor or midwife should discuss with you how to be aware of signs of preterm labor and what the procedures are for calling in if you think you're in early labor.

Signs of preterm labor to watch for include:

- Dull, low backache
- Increase in vaginal discharge
- Bleeding from the vagina
- Sudden gush of fluid from the vagina (water breaking)
- Slow, continuous trickle of fluid from the vagina
- Four or more contractions an hour
- Increase in vaginal or pelvic pressure
- Decrease in fetal movement
- Feeling that something's not right

Call your practitioner right away if you experience any of these signs of early labor. Your doctor or midwife might warn you about some other specific signs, so be sure to add these to your list and know what to do if you experience them. Don't let anyone put you off, or let your fear of bothering someone stop you from making the call.

If you experience preterm labor, it is important to follow your practitioner's instructions to the letter. This will probably include limiting your ability to exercise. He may even order bed rest for you, either at home or in the hospital. Either way, exercise at this point in pregnancy would be detrimental to your health and well-being and that of your baby. Be sure to ask any questions you have of your doctor or midwife. These are obviously not the only reasons to modify your workouts. Always talk to your doctor or midwife at each visit about your routines and how you are modifying them as your pregnancy progresses.

Exercise for the Second Trimester

During the first part of the second trimester, you won't notice much difference in how you need to do your exercises. As the trimester progresses and your abdomen begins to expand, you will notice modifications that you need to make for comfort and safety. Supine positions are an absolute no-no during your second and third trimesters because of the harmful possibilities to both your stomach muscles as well as the blood flow to the baby; modifications for supine exercises are mostly side-lying suggestions, but if you can't find a comfortable modification to a supine exercise, do not perform it!

ALERT

During the second trimester, you may be lulled into a false sense of security because the pregnancy is "old news"—and besides, you feel great! Don't let this type of attitude keep you from warming up. Remember, those hormones can add injury to insult if you do have a problem.

Things to watch for include proper clothing and ventilation to avoid overheating. To stay well hydrated, it might take more water than in the previous trimester. And general safety issues, like the shift in the center of gravity, should be noted.

Relaxation and Cool-Downs

If you've started childbirth or relaxation classes, this would be the time to try to incorporate some of those teachings into your workout. You can do some self-relaxation at the end of each cool-down period to entice your mind and to relax your body.

ESSENTIAL

Childbirth classes come in many different varieties. Choose one that is independently taught by a certified instructor. There are many organizations to choose from, including: Lamaze (*www.lamaze-childbirth .com*); ICEA (www.icea.org); and the Bradley Method (*www.bradley birth.com*). Learn about the different philosophies and find an instructor in your area.

Progressive relaxation is one great tool to use in life and in labor. Find a comfortable position for relaxing, like side-lying or semi-sitting. Beginning at the top of your head, imagine yourself releasing tension from the top of your head as you exhale. Slowly go down through all the major parts of your body, paying particular attention to your personal trouble spots for tension. Make sure to include your forehead, jaw, neck, shoulders, arms, wrists, hands, abdomen, upper and lower back, pelvis, pelvic floor, thighs, buttocks, calves, and feet. Feel free to include other parts, or even do fingers and toes individually.

CHAPTER 17

Third Trimester

In the third trimester, you are starting down the home-stretch! Your third trimester lasts from the twenty-sixth week after your last menstrual period until the birth of your baby, which usually takes place somewhere between the thirty-eighth to forty-second weeks. As with your first and second trimesters, it helps to be prepared for your last trimester by learning about the changes your body will likely go through, how your baby is developing, and what you need from your diet and exercise to keep yourself and your baby healthy and prepared for the big finale!

In Case You Didn't Know . . .

By your last trimester, you will have put on much of your pregnancy weight as your baby fully grows and develops. You should be gaining weight at a rate of about 1 pound per week. You will probably begin to feel some pain in the ribs as your baby grows and pushes upward on your rib cage. The pressure may also give you some indigestion and heartburn. You may begin to see stretch marks as your uterus expands. Your balance and mobility will also change as you get bigger. Throughout your last trimester, as your baby continues to grow, you will begin to experience some discomforts such as leg cramps, mild swelling of the feet and ankles, constipation, difficulty with sleep, shortness of breath, lower abdominal pain, backaches, and Braxton Hicks contractions. You may feel a more frequent urge to urinate again as you did in the first trimester.

FACT

Around your twenty-eighth to thirtieth week of pregnancy, or even as early as twenty weeks, you may experience episodes in which your belly tightens, becomes firm, and then relaxes. This feeling, which is very normal, comes from contractions of the uterine muscles called Braxton Hicks contractions. They are a type of warmup or practice for the uterus for labor. Braxton Hicks contractions usually occur no more than four to six times per hour in your ninth month. If you can't tell the difference between Braxton Hicks contractions and true labor contractions, ask your doctor.

All women "carry" differently. Some will carry the baby higher or lower, bigger or smaller, wider or more compact. All these depend on the size and position of your little one, your body type, and how much body weight you have gained.

By your ninth month, your weight gain should be somewhere around 24 to 29 pounds. It may get more uncomfortable to sleep and move around, and it is normal to become moody and irritable. As you near the end, you may notice alternating feelings of fatigue and bursts of energy.

It is a good time to think ahead and prepare for your return from the hospital . . . with a newborn! Use those energy bursts to start stocking your freezer with foods you can easily pop in your oven or microwave. Cook casseroles, chili, soups, and other dishes that can be frozen and prepared later when you are too busy to worry about cooking.

What's Going On

The final stretch of the pregnancy journey has finally begun. As you've learned to adapt to the physical and mental changes throughout pregnancy, the third trimester is no different. As you get closer to your due date, you may find that fatigue and insomnia once again begin to plague you. These complaints are very common for pregnant women in their third trimester due to the great changes that are taking place in their minds and bodies as they prepare for the birth of their baby. While annoying, none of these troubles are life-threatening and most of these temporary discomforts can be resolved naturally.

Keep the Swelling Down

Moderate swelling or retaining of water in the hands, face, legs, ankles, and/or feet, known as *edema*, is very normal in pregnancy. Edema is caused in pregnancy by the increase in blood volume and other fluids needed for the baby as well as from an increase in hormones. Ankles and feet tend to swell because the size of your baby and uterus can put pressure on the return circulation to your legs. The key is to get the fluids moving and to maximize the output of the kidneys. Edema can happen at any time during pregnancy, but it tends to begin around the fifth month and increase in the third trimester.

FACT

During the course of your pregnancy, your body will produce approximately 50 percent more blood and body fluids to meet the needs of your developing baby. The accumulation of these extra fluids accounts for almost 25 percent of a woman's weight gain during pregnancy.

Moderate swelling is expected and normal in pregnancy as long as it is not accompanied by an increase in blood pressure and protein in the urine, which can be a sign of preeclampsia. Sudden or severe edema can also be a sign of this condition. If you experience these noticeable symptoms, contact your doctor immediately.

Here are a few tips for minimizing any swelling during pregnancy:

- Put your feet up, and elevate your legs whenever possible. Try not to cross your legs as this only makes circulation more difficult. Any time you can, get off your feet; the blood can circulate better and not pool in the extremities.
- Dress comfortably, and avoid wearing clothes that are too restrictive or too tight. That includes shoes that are comfortable and not tight or too high-heeled.
- Wear supportive hose or stockings that are specifically designed for pregnancy. Make sure you are fitted correctly.
- Avoid standing in one place for long periods of time. Move around to keep your blood circulating. Moderate exercise such as walking and stretching can be helpful.
- Minimize your time outdoors if it is hot and humid.
- Rest by lying on your left side as much as possible, and not just at night, but several times throughout the day for about thirty minutes.
- Drink water and fluids, at least eight 8-ounce glasses per day, to help keep your kidneys functioning properly and help flush out retained fluids.
- Don't consume excessive amounts of sodium. Avoid adding salt to foods and eating too many salty snacks or heavily cured foods.
- Visit your doctor regularly so she can monitor your blood pressure and severity of fluid retention.

Coping with an Achy Back and Legs

Backaches and leg aches can be very common later in pregnancy, as the baby begins to grow larger. By the second and third trimester, the weight of the baby on the pelvic bone can compress your sciatic nerve and result in pain along your back and legs. In addition to the weight of the baby and uterus, other causes of common aches include poor posture, hormonal changes (which can cause a loosening of the ligaments), and weak abdominal muscles. It is important to practice good posture with your pelvis tucked in and your shoulders back to relieve some of the pressure.

Here are some other techniques that might help relieve backaches:

- Wear low-heeled but not flat shoes that have a good supportive arch.
- Do not lift heavy objects, such as children. If you have to lift something, bend at the knees, and keep your back straight. Use your legs to lift and not your back.
- Sit in chairs with good back support, or put a small pillow behind the lower part of your back.
- Try to sleep on your side with one or two pillows placed between your legs for support.
- Apply heat or cold to painful areas, or have someone massage them.
- Stay physically active to keep muscles toned and strong. Yoga stretches a few times a week may help relieve back pain, but make sure you learn how to correctly perform the stretches to avoid injury.
- Sleep on a firm mattress.
- Keep your weight under control with proper diet and exercise. Gain only the recommended amount of weight. Gaining too much weight will put even more stress on your legs and back.

If back and/or leg pain is very bothersome, speak to your doctor. A licensed physical therapist may be able to help you ease your pain through postural awareness and safe exercises.

Dreadful Varicose Veins

Some women may get painful varicose veins during pregnancy, particularly if this problem runs in the family. The increase in blood volume, along with changes in hormone levels, and the increasing size of the baby and uterus can all add to the likelihood of varicose veins. The veins in your legs help to transport blood back to the heart and lungs for reoxygenation. It is a tough job, though, because gravity pulls the blood downward instead of up toward the heart and lungs. The leg muscles try to fight this gravity by contracting. As the muscles contract, blood moves through the veins where valves confine and hold it. If these valves become overwhelmed, which they often do during the later months of pregnancy, blood collects and stretches the vein walls out of shape. The painful result is visually swollen varicose veins. Support pantyhose can help to ease some of the pain. Put your feet up whenever possible, and avoid standing for long periods of time. Take a brisk walk every day to increase circulation. If your varicose veins become intensely bothersome and painful, talk with your doctor about other types of treatment.

Fatigue and Insomnia

When timed appropriately, physical activity will help increase your ability to sleep. So if your problem is really a physical one, doing exercises or your fitness routine, however modified, should be done prior to the evening hours. Exercising just before bed can make sleep nearly impossible. The physical exercises can also help you address problem areas. For example, good stretches can help you alleviate and prevent backaches.

ALERT

Trying to determine if you're staying awake at night because of your mind racing or physical issues can be a tough call. But the benefits to you and your baby make the question worth asking. It can also help you solve the problems that are preventing you from getting a good night's rest.

If you determine that the cause of your wakefulness is more mental and emotional, the relaxation exercises you can do will often help you learn to put these thoughts out of your mind. Training your mind to focus on certain topics will also be beneficial in labor. The ability to focus internally and deal with the need at hand is very useful. That's not to say you shouldn't address issues and concerns—just don't do it at bedtime.

ESSENTIAL

Dreams as a part of pregnancy are often hard to shake. While some may be funny, others may be your way of expressing your worst fears about parenting. Either way, keeping a dream journal next to your bed to write down your dreams can help you deal with them when you're awake.

While medications may not be useful in trying to help you turn in at night, there are other things to try. Old remedies like a warm bath (but not too warm) and a good book really can help. Sometimes practicing your labor relaxation just before bed can make it easier to fall asleep. Even the proverbial glass of milk can be helpful.

Return of Nausea

Feeling nauseated is enough to make anyone want to lie in bed all day. Unfortunately for some women, the return of nausea and vomiting in the third trimester is a reality. Be prepared to deal with it should it rear its ugly head again.

The cause of the nausea and vomiting is thought to be partially hormonal, as it was in your first trimester. However, the third trimester brings about a new issue—the baby. Sometimes the pressure of the baby's growing body and the expanding uterus on your other organs is enough to cause your stomach to be upset.

You might find that eating smaller meals will help you avoid some of these issues. You also need to try eating more frequently to make up for the smaller meals. This ensures that you and the baby are still getting adequate nutrition.

Heartburn

You might also find that nausea and vomiting are connected with heartburn. Heartburn is what you call it when you experience a burning sensation in your esophagus. It is caused from the relaxation of the sphincter muscle that guards the stomach. The relaxation is caused by the hormones of pregnancy.

FACT

Papaya enzymes can help alleviate pain and irritation from heartburn. You can try eating papaya fruit, drinking papaya juice, or even taking papaya tablets. These enzymes help with digestion.

When you experience this relaxation of the sphincter muscle, stomach acids are able to leak out of the stomach and into the esophagus. This is what causes the irritation. At the end of your pregnancy, the growing uterus also places a lot of pressure on your organs. This can also encourage the escape of stomach acids into the esophagus. The good news is that there are many things you can do to help with the pain and even elimination of heartburn:

- Eat smaller meals.
- Remain upright after you eat.
- Avoid greasy or spicy foods.
- Avoid foods that seem to bring on heartburn.
- Eat more frequently throughout the day and evening.
- Try a glass of milk, a teaspoon of honey, or TUMS to help alleviate pain.

What's Happening with Baby?

During your last trimester, your baby continues to grow larger, and his body organs continue to mature. Your baby is completing his development for his introduction to the world. With your baby growing and getting heavier, the last three months can get a bit uncomfortable—just keep thinking about the end result!

Your Seventh Month (26 to 30 Weeks)

Your baby will really start squirming around between the twenty-seventh and thirty-second weeks. Starting with your seventh month, the baby's lungs continue to develop, but they are not yet fully mature. To practice waking up Mom and Dad at all hours of the night, the baby begins to develop patterns of waking and sleeping. The baby's hands are active, and fingernails are growing. Muscle coordination is getting much better. The baby can now suck her thumb and can even cry. By week twenty-eight, the baby's eyelids are opening. The lungs are developed enough that if the baby were born prematurely, she would have a good chance at survival but would need to stay in a neonatal intensive care unit (NICU). As your seventh month progresses and the baby grows larger, he experiences a harder time moving around in the uterus due to space constraints. However, he still seems to find the room to do some kicking and stretching. The baby gains more fat on his body to help control his own temperature.

By the end of this month, the eyebrows and eyelashes are filled in and any hair the baby has on his head is becoming thicker. The head is now proportioned to the rest of the body. The baby's hearing is fully developed, and she can respond to stimuli such as pain, light, and sounds. Toward the end of this month amniotic fluid begins to diminish. Your baby now measures about seventeen inches from head to toe and weighs about 2 to 4 pounds.

ALERT

Around the seventh month of your pregnancy, it is normal for your blood pressure to increase slightly. However, you should contact your doctor if you experience severe headaches, blurred vision, or severe swelling in your hands, feet, and/or ankles. These specific symptoms could signal the beginning of a condition called preeclampsia, which is pregnancy-induced hypertension, or high blood pressure.

Your Eighth Month (31 to 34 Weeks)

Starting with your eighth month, the baby is becoming too big to move easily inside the uterus. It may seem that the baby is moving less. The baby is developing more fat beneath his thin layer of skin, and he's starting to practice opening his eyes. Most of his internal systems and organs are now well developed except the lungs, which are not quite yet fully matured. The baby's brain continues to develop at a rapid pace. These weeks mark a ton of growth for the baby. During the last seven weeks, the baby gains more than half his birth weight. As the baby becomes larger, he begins to run out of room and takes the fetal position by curling up. By the end of the eighth month, the baby begins to move into a head-down position, although that may not be his final position at birth. Your baby now measures around 19.8 inches from head to toe and weighs about 5 pounds.

Your Ninth Month (35 to 40 Weeks)

By nine months, your baby's lungs are almost fully developed. She still doesn't have quite enough fat under the skin to keep herself warm outside of the womb, but she is working on it. By the ninth month, the baby begins to drop lower into your abdomen, usually with the head in a downward position. The brain has been rapidly developing, and the baby's reflexes are coordinated so she can blink her eyes, turn her head, grasp firmly with her hands, and respond to stimuli. Every day, the baby is taking on a rounder shape, developing pinker skin, and losing her wrinkled appearance. The baby is beginning to get antibodies from you that will help protect her from illness.

In this last month, the growth of your baby tends to slow down, yet he is still collecting fat under his skin and, therefore, putting on more weight. The toenails have grown to the tips of the toes, as have the fingernails, which have grown to the tips of the fingers. The baby's arm and leg muscles are stronger, and he is beginning to practice breathing and working out his lungs. By the end of the ninth month, your baby will drop farther into your pelvis, hopefully with head aimed downward to the birth canal, to prepare for delivery. The drop of the baby will help you breathe a little easier. Your baby's length at birth is about eighteen to twenty inches on average, and she weighs about 7.5 pounds. Length and weight vary greatly from baby to baby.

What Your Body Needs

Of course, good nutrition and proper weight gain are also essential during your third trimester. Too little or too much weight gain can become a more significant problem in this homestretch. Calcium intake is also crucial because the baby's bones are developing rapidly during the last trimester.

Weight: Walking a Thin Line

During these last three months, you can go either way when it comes to weight. The weight of your baby is increasing rapidly. For some women, this might mean that at meals, you feel fuller faster, making it difficult to get the essential calories that are still needed. If that's the case, it is best to try to eat smaller meals more often throughout the day. Snacks in between meals can help boost calorie intake. Choose a variety of snacks that will supply the nutrients that you need. If you have not gained enough weight throughout your entire pregnancy, you may not be able to make up for it all in the last trimester, but you can begin to ensure you are getting all of the calories that you need for a normal-weight baby.

The flip side of the coin is gaining too much weight. You should be gaining about 1 pound per week during the third trimester. But by the ninth month, it is really the baby who is plumping up and not you. This is a good thing because the baby needs to be at a healthy weight by delivery. Low birthweight babies have a harder time thriving and are much more susceptible to health and developmental problems. If by this time you are concerned that you have gained too much weight, discuss it with your doctor. If you feel you are gaining too much weight, do *not* restrict your caloric intake in hopes of losing a few pounds before the birth of your baby. In your ninth month, it is still important to eat a healthy diet and to pack a nutritional punch at each and every meal and snack. It is never too late to switch to a healthier diet for the proper nourishment of your baby and for a healthier weight gain. Eating a healthier diet can also help provide you with the important energy you will need for the delivery process.

Crucial Calcium

Although calcium is an essential nutrient before, during, and after pregnancy, it is especially crucial in the last three months of pregnancy. This is the time that your baby's bones and teeth are rapidly developing. If the baby can't get enough calcium from your dietary intake, he will take what he needs from your own stores. If your baby is relying on your stores of calcium for his needs, this can be detrimental to your health in the long run—for instance, by increasing your risk of osteoporosis. For this reason, it is vital that you get plenty of calcium through food and supplements in this critical third trimester.

Keep in mind that you can always overdo too much of a good thing, so watch that you don't abuse calcium supplements. You should not get more than 2,500 mg of calcium per day.

Exercising: Fitness for the Finale

As with the first and second trimesters, there are specific things going on this trimester that you need to be aware of as you work out. Be sure to inform your practitioner about your exercise regimen at every visit to ensure you're both on the same page, and he is well aware of your abilities and experience with improved strength and stamina throughout your pregnancy.

Most of the time, there are no specific recommendations to stop exercising prior to labor. Many women go through pregnancy exercising until the day of labor without a single issue. Other moms might feel tired and worn out, decreasing their workouts in intensity and frequency as they go. Either way is fine as long as it's what is right for you and your baby.

The precautions for exercising in the third trimester include watching for signs of preterm labor, dehydration, safety issues, and symptoms of maternal supine hypotension syndrome. If you have any complications from these or other things that arise in your workout, stop exercising immediately. Call your doctor or midwife to discuss possible modifications.

Keep in Mind . . .

As you finish up the last months of your pregnancy, there are probably a million things on your mind (and to-do list!). Keep in mind that, while you're in the homestretch of your pregnancy and preparing for the birth, you are still very pregnant and not able to do as much as you'd probably like. "Nesting" may kick your energy levels into overdrive here and there, but your body's new shape, size, and conservation of energy should give you enough reason to take things a little more slowly to prevent any injuries, preterm labor, or just plain overwhelming and stressful feelings.

Clumsiness and Lack of Motivation

If you thought you were clumsy last trimester, just wait! Your bulging belly is beautiful, but it can also cause you to take unnecessary spills if you're not careful. Wear sensible shoes, and watch for hazards, such as wet floors.

ESSENTIAL

If you feel like taking time off but really don't want to, consider modifying your workout. Perhaps you can do a warmup and cool-down, rather than the entire workout. Maybe it's time for a change in your workout. Rather than doing your aerobics today, go for a swim instead.

The third trimester might also be one when you have days of not wanting to do much of anything. Or you might want to divert your energies into preparing your baby's space in your home. Either way, it's okay to take days off. Remember that motivation will come and go, particularly in this third trimester. Your mind will wander and you'll have other things to focus on. Give yourself the space to take time off.

Feeling Overwhelmed

Feeling overwhelmed can also play a big part in lack of motivation. You've got the pregnancy and impending birth on your mind. Perhaps you're concerned about your job, or maybe you've even taken other big plunges, like a new home or other investments. These all weigh heavily on you when trying to focus. A change in pace or activity can help.

FACT

The confidence you've gained from your fitness routines and the strength in your body will give you confidence and faith for labor, birth, and parenting. Remember to draw on these strengths as you go forward.

Learning to Slow Down

As your pregnancy draws near the end, you are probably learning that taking things a bit more easily is wise. Sometimes your body forces you to take it easy. Other times it's the natural progression of the cycle of pregnancy.

No matter why you decide to slow down or when, in the third trimester, it's important to recognize this as a good thing. Easing up on your fitness routines gives your body a chance to finish the pregnancy and prepare for labor, birth, and postpartum.

Preparing for Labor and Delivery

Your strong mind and body, which you've spent the last nine months or more preparing for this grand adventure, will not fail you. Remember to listen to the signals as you have done throughout your pregnancy fitness sessions. Follow your body's lead and be prepared to go with the flow. Mind and body, and flexibility and knowledge will go a long way toward making your labor and birth experience a great one to remember for the rest of your life.

CHAPTER 18

Labor and Delivery

Even if you've read everything ever written about labor and delivery, taken copious notes in childbirth class, watched hours of birth stories on cable TV, and questioned all your friends on their birth experiences, you'll still find your labor is different in some way from that of others. Because every woman's labor is unique, comparisons of length, progress, and pain perception can be inaccurate and even discouraging. Follow your own path, and you'll do fine.

Contractions

The first signal of labor is contractions—the tightening and release of your uterus that helps propel your baby down the birth canal. These contractions are different from the Braxton Hicks ones you've possibly had in that they occur at regular intervals, are painful, and are slowly but surely opening the door (that is, the cervix) for baby's exit.

You don't need to rush to the hospital or birthing center after your first contraction. But you should call your doctor or midwife to let her know labor has started and how far apart contractions are. Remember, contractions are timed from the beginning of one to the start of the next. Your provider will let you know at what point you should head for the hospital or birthing center. Until then, you can labor in the comfort and privacy of your own home. However, if the pain from contractions starts to be more than you can handle without professional help, have your coach call your provider back and let her know you're heading for the hospital early.

At the Hospital or Birthing Center

When you do arrive at your birthing center or hospital, the nursing staff will prep (prepare) you for labor and delivery. While the prepping process varies with each facility's policy and doctor's preference, there are some common steps you can know about beforehand.

- **Suit Up.** You'll change into your hospital gown or nightgown from home. Try not to wear a lot of jewelry or other extraneous items that can get lost in the shuffle from room to room.
- **The Enema Within.** While it's *not* very common in today's hospitals or birth facilities, it's possible that your hospital may require an enema to clear out your bowel so that baby will have a smoother passage down the neighboring birth canal. Find out in advance if this is required; you might be able to administer it at home if it makes you more comfortable. If contractions have had you on the toilet all day and you've got nothing left to give, let your nurse know and staff might bypass this step.

- **Drop a Line.** Your nurse may insert a needle with a heparin lock and secure it to your arm with surgical tape. If intravenous (IV) medication is suddenly needed during labor, it can be easily hooked up. Other hospitals will hook you up to an IV line as a matter of course and administer a glucose solution to keep you hydrated. Other medications can be added to the line as necessary.

- **Baby Monitor.** Chances are good that you've experienced the fetal and uterine monitors during a visit to your provider, so this part of the procedure should be familiar to you. The monitor will give you a visible and audible look at your contractions and the fetal heart rate; it will allow you and your coach to see when a contraction is coming and, more important, when it seems to be almost over. It will also pick up fetal heart sounds and alert you to any stress the baby may be experiencing from oxygen deprivation or problems with the umbilical cord. An internal monitor might be used if you are considered to be at high risk.

Natural Pain Relief Options for Home and Hospital

In early labor when contractions are getting intense but are still not close enough to leave for the hospital, there are a few ways you can ease the pain.

ESSENTIAL

If you don't want to be bound to your bed during labor, find out whether your birth facility has fetal monitors that use telemetry. These wireless monitors strap on like a regular external device so that you don't have to remain plugged into anything. There are even telemetry units that are waterproof, if you plan on easing labor pains with hydrotherapy.

A Comfortable Position

At home, or at the hospital, it's a good idea to have plenty of pillows on hand. Wherever you choose to do most of your laboring, you can experiment with different positions, such as on all fours, against a wall, and leaning against someone or something while bent forward at the waist in order to find a position that's most comfortable for you.

Back Labor

Back labor, which occurs when baby's face is toward your abdomen rather than toward your spine, can cause severe lower-back pain. Ask your partner to try massage or a warm water bottle to ease contractions. The soothing jets of a whirlpool tub can do wonders, if you have one. If your water has broken, however, never take a soak without approval from your provider.

Stress Down, Positivity Up

Keep positive, supportive people around you. Let your coach be your buffer and clear out any distractions. Try to remain focused on riding through and past the contraction. Fix your eyes on something that relaxes you and practice the breathing exercises you learned in childbirth class to keep the oxygen and blood flowing. Don't hyperventilate. Talk or groan through the peak of the contraction if it helps.

It's difficult to relax while you're in the midst of a really big, really uncomfortable contraction. However, letting go in between contractions can help ease your mind and body and loosen you up for impending delivery. You probably learned a few relaxation exercises in childbirth class. If so, now is the time to try them, as they can make the pain more manageable.

Progressive Relaxation

Performing a series of muscle tightening and releasing, referred to as "progressive relaxation," is a good way to release your stress. Make sure you're in comfortable clothes in a soothing atmosphere (that is, quiet and perhaps dim). Recline with your head and back elevated, then start tensing and releasing each muscle group, from your head to your toes. Breathe in with the tension, and blow out with the release. Try to clear your head of everything but the sensation at hand. If you practice this prior to labor, it can be a good tool for managing some of the early pain when contractions are still relatively far apart.

Pharmaceutical Pain Relief Options

Once you arrive at the hospital, you will have analgesics and anesthetics available for pain relief, if you choose to use them.

Analgesics

Analgesics deaden the pain by depressing your nervous system. They make you sleepy and help you rest between contractions. The analgesics Demerol (meperidine), Stadol (butorphanol), Nubain (nalbuphine), and Sublimaze (fentanyl) are commonly used in labor. Although some of these drugs, such as Demerol, can even allow you to nap between contractions, you remain conscious under their influence (albeit a bit giddy). Although these medications can cross the placenta, when they are properly administered in the appropriate dosages they should not cause baby any serious side effects.

ESSENTIAL

Pain relief in labor was roundly condemned for many centuries, partly on biblical grounds (think Eve and the apple), until Queen Victoria of England requested and was administered chloroform for the birth of her eighth and ninth children. The resultant births of Prince Leopold and Princess Beatrice were attended by a pioneer in anesthetic use, Dr. John Snow.

General Anesthesia

You may also receive either a general or local (regional) anesthetic. General anesthesia brings about a complete loss of consciousness ("puts you to sleep"). General anesthesia is rarely used in labor and delivery, usually only in cases of an emergency cesarean section when there isn't adequate time to prep the patient with a local anesthetic. Newborns arriving under the influence of a general anesthesia can be drowsy and slow to respond due to the effects of the anesthesia.

Local Anesthesia

Local anesthesia, also called regional anesthesia, numbs only a specific portion of the body and leaves you awake and alert. The most commonly used local anesthesia is probably the lumbar epidural. Injected into the space between two vertebrae of your lower back (in the epidural space), this type of anesthesia is administered when you are well into labor; it will temporarily numb the nerves all the way from your belly button to your knees. An epidural takes twenty minutes to start working and can lower your blood pressure, so you'll be put on the fetal monitor and hooked up to an IV fluid drip if you're given an epidural.

FACT

A spinal block is similar to an epidural in that it's administered in the lower back. However, a spinal is delivered directly into your lower spine, not into the spaces between your vertebrae as in an epidural. Used right at delivery only or during a C-section, the spinal will numb you from your rib cage all the way down.

Some providers may require you to wait until you reach a certain dilation benchmark or stage of labor to have an epidural. But if you are being induced, an epidural might be in order earlier because you can experience a lot of pain before there is any major progress in the dilation of your cervix. With an epidural most providers will give you more time to push because your sensation is impaired. If you have concerns about epidural timing, discuss them with your health care provider.

The epidural is administered through a small plastic catheter in your back. An anesthesiologist will place the epidural catheter and administer the local anesthetic agent. Before he starts, your lower back will be draped and the insertion spot swabbed with antiseptic or iodine. You might be asked to pull your knees and chin toward your chest so that your spine is more visible. The catheter is inserted in the space between the fourth and fifth vertebrae, and the anesthesia injected. You may feel a slight stinging sensation down your legs, but your breathing and the involuntary muscles working those contractions won't be affected. The insertion of an epidural catheter allows anesthetics to be administered on an as-needed basis and is useful should a C-section be required.

When insertion is complete, the doctor will secure the catheter and you can get comfortable again. Watch the fetal monitor for the start of the next contraction. You'll be amazed at how what was turning you inside out a moment ago is barely perceptible now. The numbness will take several hours to wear off and may restrict your movements during the birth, but an epidural can be a great pain management tool.

Women who want the pain relief benefits of an epidural but also wish to retain the ability to move around during labor are candidates for a low-dose combination spinal epidural, sometimes referred to as a walking epidural. An epidural catheter is inserted, and an injection of a narcotic is administered into the spinal fluid using a smaller needle that fits through the epidural catheter. A walking epidural is usually faster acting than a conventional epidural and allows you to retain enough sensation to move and walk, which can speed the labor process.

One, Two, Three, Push!

Labor is a series of three distinct stages, aptly called first, second, and third stages. For most women the longest span is the first stage, which lasts from the earliest signs of labor right through baby's descent into the birth canal, in preparation for stage two—pushing. Stage three consists of delivering the placenta; mothers usually feel this is a cakewalk after all the hard work involved in baby's arrival.

First Stage

The first stage of labor begins with early (latent) labor and ends with active labor. Your provider probably uses the term transition (descent) to refer to the end of first-stage labor.

During the early phase the cervix effaces (thins) and dilates (opens). This ripening process perhaps started several weeks ago, well before the regular contractions of early labor began. Now your cervix will dilate to about 4 or 5 centimeters. Contractions will arrive every 5 to 10 minutes and last 60 to 90 seconds. If your partner or coach isn't around, now is the time to contact him so that he can be by your side. Then touch base with your provider, who will tell you at what point you should head to the hospital or birthing facility.

Try to stay up and moving through contractions as much as you can to let gravity help your baby descend. Consider a light liquid snack (for example, broth or juice) to power up your energy reserves for the long road ahead. Rest if possible. Try the breathing and relaxation techniques you picked up in childbirth class as well as the coach-assisted massage or showering to get you through these first few hours. Then leave for the hospital and the next phase—active labor.

In active labor your contractions are coming closer together regularly, perhaps 3 to 5 minutes apart, and they can be intense, lasting 45 to 60 seconds. These strong contractions are dilating your cervix from about 4 or 5 centimeters to around 8.

Once you reach the birthing center or hospital, you'll be quickly prepped as described earlier and given an internal exam to check the dilation of your cervix. The baby's position will be checked, and you will probably be hooked up to a fetal monitor to assess the baby's well-being.

Other signs that active labor is in progress:

- **Your membranes rupture.** If the amniotic sac hasn't already broken, it will now or very soon.
- **You bleed from your vagina.** More of the mucus plug is being expelled.
- **You need air.** Put those cleansing breaths and other breathing techniques into practice. Your hard-working uterus needs oxygen.
- **Your back really hurts.** The baby's head is pushing on your backbone. Massage can help.
- **You have muscle cramps.** Again, massage can help the ill-timed charley horse.
- **You're exhausted and physically spent.** Remember what you're working toward. Let your coach know how you're feeling so that she can motivate you and get you whatever she can to keep you moving forward.

Don't feel inadequate or guilty about asking for pain medication at any point if you want it. You wouldn't hesitate to take Novocain if you were getting a wisdom tooth pulled, yet having an 8-pound child pulled through a 10-centimeter opening doesn't qualify? Pain medication is a tool, just like your breathing exercises. Wisely used, it can result in a better birth experience for both you and your child.

Once your cervix reaches 8 centimeters and contractions start coming one on top of another to get you to full dilation, the end of the first stage (transition) has arrived. Because of the frequency of contractions and the overwhelming urge to push, this is the most difficult part of labor. Fortunately, it culminates in your child's delivery, once you bridge those final 2 centimeters to become fully dilated.

As you begin to transition from first- to second-stage labor:

- You can become nauseated and may even vomit.
- You have chills or sweats, and your muscles twitch.
- Your back really, really hurts.
- Contractions are just minutes apart, if even that.
- There is pressure in your rectum from the baby.
- You are absolutely exhausted.
- You may feel like pushing even though your cervix is not yet fully dilated.

Although every fiber of your body is probably screaming "PUSH!," you need to hold back just a few moments more. Your cervix is almost, but not quite, open far enough for baby's safe passage. Take quick, shallow breaths and resist the urge to push until your doctor or midwife gives the go-ahead.

ESSENTIAL

If your birthing center or hospital has whirlpool tubs or showers available for laboring moms, you might find the pulsating water welcome relief for getting through contractions. This pain relief method (called hydrotherapy) is not the same as a water birth, in which a baby is actually born submerged in a pool of water.

Second Stage, or *Push!*

Your cervix has made it to 10 centimeters, and you are finally allowed to push. This second stage can last anywhere from a few minutes (with second or subsequent babies) to several hours. Your contractions will still arrive regularly, but they aren't quite as close together—a welcome relief. Pushing is very hard work, but the sensations may change from the intense gripping you've experienced to more of a stinging or burning sensation.

ESSENTIAL

If possible, try to find a pushing position that makes you feel comfortable and in control. Use gravity to your advantage by kneeling, squatting, or sitting up with your legs and knees spread far apart. Stirrups are likely available, but don't feel forced into using them if they don't work for you.

Your birth attendant and/or coach will let you know when the peak of the contraction occurs, the optimum time for pushing effectively. Use whatever it takes to push effectively. If that means moaning, grunting, and emitting other primal sounds that make your prenatal snoring sound like a lullaby by comparison, go for it. The people attending your birth have probably heard just about everything. Don't be embarrassed, because the noise won't even faze them.

The emergence of the head at your vaginal opening starts with a small patch of skin visible during the peak of a push. The patch may recede when you rest but will reappear at the next contraction. Unless your baby is arriving in a breech position, the head will finally crown (bulge) right out of your vaginal opening. You may be asked to stop pushing momentarily as the baby's head is ready to emerge, in order to prevent perineal tearing. Panting can help you suppress the urge. The obstetrician or midwife may decide on an episiotomy if your skin doesn't appear willing to stretch another millimeter, or she may attempt perineal massage.

Finally the head slides face down past the perineum and is eased out carefully by the birth attendant to prevent injury to the baby. The attendant may wipe the eyes, nose, and mouth and suction any mucus or fluid from her upper respiratory tract. It's all downhill from here as the rest of the body slides out.

As your baby leaves the quiet, dim warmth of the womb for the bright lights and big noises of the outside world, his respiratory reflexes kick in and the newborn lungs fill with air for the first time. He'll probably test out those lungs with a full-fledged wail. Your doctor will place the baby on your stomach for introductions, usually with the umbilical cord still attached.

The cord will continue to pulse with blood flow for a few minutes. The timing of the actual clamping and severing of the cord will depend upon your practitioner, and this is a matter of some debate in childbirth circles. Some professionals believe that waiting until pulsation has stopped or even until after the placenta is delivered improves baby's circulation and blood pressure, reducing baby's risk of early childhood anemia and mom's chance of hemorrhage. Other practitioners still follow the traditional method of clamping and cutting the cord earlier. You may want to talk the issue over with your doctor in advance of delivery day if you have concerns about the timing of the cord cut. If baby requires resuscitation, or if the cord is tightly wrapped around a body part or is exceedingly short, it will be cut sooner.

Most practitioners will give dad (or even mom) the option of cutting the cord in an uncomplicated birth. Don't feel bad if it isn't your cup of tea, especially if either one of you is a bit squeamish. Better to spend the time cuddling your baby than being picked up off the delivery room floor.

FACT

A 2006 Cochrane Review found that delayed clamping of the umbilical cord for preterm infants may improve health outcomes. Among preemies who had a delay in cord clamping of anywhere from 30 seconds to 2 minutes, the risk of intraventricular hemorrhage (bleeding on the brain) and the need for postpartum transfusion were significantly reduced.

Some parents choose to bank their child's umbilical cord blood and/or placenta blood after birth. This blood contains stem cells, those miraculous little blank slates from which all organs and tissues are built. Cord and/or placenta blood collected immediately after birth is placed in a collection kit and flown to a facility where it is cryogenically frozen and banked for later use, if needed. The theory behind banking this at birth is that if your child ever develops a disease or condition requiring stem-cell treatment, the blood can be thawed and used for her treatment. If it matches certain biological markers, it may be used to treat other family members as well. However, banking is cost prohibitive for many and requires an ongoing annual storage fee. You will need to make arrangements for this before your delivery day.

Third Stage, or You Aren't Done Yet!

The third stage of labor is the delivery of the placenta. The entire placenta must be expelled to prevent bleeding and infection complications later on. Contractions will continue, and your doctor may press down on your abdomen and massage your uterus or tug gently on the end of the umbilical cord hanging from your vagina. You might also be injected with the hormone Pitocin (oxytocin) to step up your contractions and expel the placenta. You'll be given pushing directives again, but this part will seem like a piece of cake given the task you've just completed.

Once the placenta is out, any stitches you require to repair tearing or episiotomy incisions will be put in. A local anesthetic will be injected to deaden the area if you aren't still anesthetized from an epidural.

Cesarean Section

A cesarean birth will be scheduled for you if you have a breech baby or other complications or conditions that indicate the need for such. It may also be performed in emergency situations in which the fetus is in distress. A cesarean is major abdominal surgery and carries with it all the risks of infection and complication that any surgical procedure does. On the positive side, with a planned C-section, the date your physician schedules the procedure is your due date, and no contractions are necessary unless you begin to labor before that time.

Before the Surgery

If you have any advance warning about your C-section, you'll probably be offered an epidural or spinal rather than general anesthesia. Before the procedure begins, you'll be prepped. A nurse may shave the area of the incision, and your arm will be hooked up to an intravenous line to receive fluids as well as pain medication. You may also be asked to drink an antacid solution called sodium citrate to neutralize your stomach acid.

Before the procedure begins, you will have a catheter inserted into your bladder. The anesthetic block will give you little control over the muscles that control urine flow, so the catheter will do the work for you, both during and after the procedure. Catheter insertion can be uncomfortable, so ask that it be inserted after you've received your anesthetic block (which will likely be in the operating room).

ESSENTIAL

If you are having a scheduled cesarean, try to arrange a few moments to consult with the anesthesiologist ahead of time. If you've had any poor experiences with anesthesia in prior C-sections, let her know so that you can improve the outcome this time around. She can also answer any questions you might have about her part of the procedure.

Ready to Roll

Once you're prepped, you will be wheeled to the operating room. In the operating room, the anesthesiologist will have you roll on your side and pull your knees toward your chest (or sit on the edge of the table with your legs hanging off) while he inserts a fine needle and catheter for an epidural or spinal block into your back. You'll then be asked to lie flat on your back with your arms straight out to the sides. A curtain just a few feet high will be positioned at your chest to keep the surgical field (the area where all the action is) sterile. This will also block your view of the procedure, so if you're determined to see baby the moment she emerges, you will want to ask for an appropriately placed mirror as early as possible.

Your arms may be loosely fastened down with Velcro straps. This is not to keep you from jumping off the table but to prevent any accidental movements that could breech the sterility of the surgical field.

The most uncomfortable part of the C-section procedure is arguably the flat-on-your-back part. It's quite possible you will become nauseated as your heavy uterus compresses your vena cava and starts to lower your blood pressure. In addition, the anesthetic itself may cause your blood pressure to fall. Although the anesthesiologist will administer medication to control this drop (called hypotension), you may get sick to your stomach. Think how long you can tolerate lying flat on your back at nine months pregnant, and you'll see why. The discomfort is compounded by the fact that you will have to vomit lying down with your head turned to the side. This is where a well-placed mate, tray in hand, is indispensable. If this does happen, hang in there and remember this part will likely be short-lived.

The obstetrician will make an incision, and the baby's head, perfectly round because she hasn't done battle with the birth canal, will be lifted out first and her mouth and nose suctioned. As your doctor helps your baby out of the incision, you'll feel a strange pulling sensation. Once the cord is cut, you'll be able to finally see your baby, albeit briefly, before she is taken for assessment and a quick cleanup by the nursing staff. In some cases the pediatric team will be in the operating room to assess the baby immediately. Your incision will be stitched closed, and you'll be wheeled off to the recovery room where your little one will meet up with you once again. The entire surgical procedure will only take about 30 to 45 minutes.

ALERT

A postdural puncture headache or spinal headache is a potential side effect of spinal blocks and epidurals. It's caused by the change in spinal fluid pressure that occurs if fluid leaks out into the epidural space following the procedure. When rest and fluids don't help, an injection of blood into the epidural space (a blood patch) may be required to ease the pain.

The Ever-Possible Emergency C-Section

If your C-section is performed under emergency circumstances, events could move quickly and you'll have fewer options. You could also be given a general anesthetic that will make you unconscious. Most dads are asked to step outside once general anesthesia has been administered, but you might want to talk to your doctor about special circumstances during childbirth.

You're a Mom!

The pinnacle of nine months of physical chaos and emotional oscillation, of queasy stomach, lost car keys, aches, pains, and hair-trigger laughter and tears, has arrived. Your baby is here, placed skin to skin to feel his mother's outside warmth for the very first time.

Meeting Baby

A thousand different feelings and emotions, from utter exhaustion to indescribable joy, will flood you as you look down at that little scrunched face, still adjusting to his new waterless environment. Wrapped in a blanket with a little stocking cap to keep his head warm, he looks so perfect yet so vulnerable.

Breastfeeding

If you're planning on breastfeeding, you can nurse him while you get acquainted, even in the recovery room if you've had a C-section. It's awe-inspiring how he knows just what to do, instinctively rooting for your breast with his eyes barely open and then latching on. Spend as long as you want getting familiar, and let baby's daddy share in the bonding, too. This is a precious time for your new family.

Baby's First Checkup

After you've met your child, she'll need some initial tests and treatments to ensure a healthy welcome into the world. The first is an Apgar test, which is simply an assessment of baby's reactivity, health, and appearance at birth. Created by noted pediatrician Dr. Virginia Apgar, the Apgar measures Appearance (skin color), Pulse, Grimace (reflexes), Activity, and Respiration. The Apgar is given just 1 minute after birth and again 5 minutes after that. The attendant will assign a score of 0 to 2 for each category and add the numbers together for the total Apgar. An average score is 7 to 10.

After the Apgar, your newborn will be measured, weighed, and have prints taken of her feet and fingers. Silver nitrate or antibiotic eye drops or ointment may be put in her eyes to prevent infection from anything she encountered in the birth canal. She'll also receive a vitamin K injection to prevent bleeding problems and a heel-stick blood draw to test for phenylketonuria (PKU), hypothyroidism, and a variety of other medical issues (screenings vary by the state your child is born in). Further tests may be administered if you have a chronic illness or have experienced complications during pregnancy. If you have diabetes, for example, your newborn will have her blood glucose (sugar) levels tested. The American Academy of Pediatrics also recommends that all infants get a hearing test and receive a hepatitis B vaccine before leaving the hospital.

Postpartum Mom

After the birth you'll have some assistance cleaning up and will be given a good supply of super-absorbent sanitary pads. You'll also be provided with a peri bottle, a plastic squirt bottle used to cleanse and soothe your perineal area with warm water each time you use the bathroom.

ALERT

If bleeding is soaking more than a pad an hour for more than three hours, let your provider know. It could be a sign that a piece of placenta is still retained in your uterus. This condition usually requires surgical removal of the placental fragments, a procedure called curettage.

Bleeding

You'll be expelling lochia for up to six weeks following birth, whether you've had a vaginal birth or a C-section. Lochia—a mixture of blood, mucus, and tissue that comes from the implantation site of the placenta—will be quite heavy in the days immediately following the birth, so don't be alarmed.

The C-Section Mom

If you've had a C-section, you'll spend some time in the recovery area before heading to your hospital room. Your incision will be checked regularly, and pain medication will be administered as needed. The next day you'll be encouraged to walk as soon as possible to get your digestive tract active again, and you'll be asked about your gas and bathroom habits ad nauseum. The nursing staff is just trying to ensure that everything is returning to normal in gastrointestinal land.

Episiotomy Care

Women who are given episiotomies will take sitz baths (also known as hip baths) to relieve pain, promote healing, and keep the area clean. A sitz bath is a small, shallow tub of water, sometimes with medication added, that you sit in. Some mild pain relievers may also be prescribed to ease episiotomy pain.

Calm Your Mind

Mortified by the possibility of losing control—both physically and emotionally—during labor? Childbirth is hard, painful work, and you need to work through it in your own way. The people around you are medical professionals and know this. Pain—in addition to the ultimate goal of meeting your child—is a great motivator for getting past feelings of fear or bashfulness.

Many women who were previously shy or self-conscious about their bodies find that pregnancy and motherhood pretty much eradicate any lingering traces of modesty. When you're in labor, you don't care if the attending doctor is animal, vegetable, or mineral; your mind and body are entirely focused on the impending arrival of your child. After they've been through the birth experience, many women find that there's virtually nothing that can embarrass them.

CHAPTER 19

Breast or Bottle?

Good nutrition for your little one right from the start will get him off to a healthy beginning. Breast milk or formula is the only food your infant needs for his first four to six months of life. If you decide to breastfeed, following some sound nutritional guidelines can ensure you are getting all of the calories and nutrients needed to nourish your baby properly.

Why Breastfeed?

One of the very first decisions new parents make is how to feed their newborn. Many health professionals agree that the ideal method is breastfeeding, though for some women this is not the best choice for physical, health, or personal reasons. For some mothers, breastfeeding is an easy transition. For others it may take some time and patience before the process is a smooth one. It is perfectly normal for it to take some time and practice. A lactation consultant should visit you in the hospital to help you get started.

FACT

The American Dietetic Association (ADA) and the American Academy of Pediatrics (AAP) both recommend that babies be breastfed exclusively for the first four to six months of life and then breastfed with complementary foods for at least twelve months.

Benefits of Breastfeeding

Even though breastfeeding is not your only option, there are many benefits to using this method to nourish your newborn in the beginning. Breastfeeding can aid in the physical, emotional, and practical needs of both the baby and the mother. Other benefits include these:

- The infant is able to eat on demand without any trouble. When the infant is hungry, the milk is ready instantly without any measuring, mixing, or warming of bottles.
- There is no concern over proper sterilization.
- Breast milk is easy for babies to digest, so there is less spitting up.
- Breast milk is rich in antibodies that can help protect the baby from intestinal, ear, urinary, and lower respiratory-tract infections, as well as pneumonia.
- If breastfeeding is continued through at least the first six months of life, it can help decrease the risk of the baby's developing food allergies.
- In babies with a family history of food allergies, breastfeeding can help lower the risk of developing asthma and some skin conditions.

- The quality and the quantity of fat in breast milk tends to be more nutritious than the fat found in most formulas.
- Breastfeeding is less expensive than formula feeding.
- New studies indicate that breastfed infants may be less likely to become obese later in life and therefore less likely to develop diabetes.
- Women who breastfeed usually return to their pre-pregnancy weight more quickly, and the uterus also returns to its normal size more quickly.
- Breastfeeding can help reduce the risk of ovarian cancer and, in pre-menopausal women, breast cancer.

How the Body Produces Breast Milk

During pregnancy, the body naturally begins to prepare itself for breastfeeding. In the first few days after birth, a woman's body produces a fluid called colostrum. This is the first milk that the infant receives. Colostrum is a thick, yellowish substance that is produced just prior to the flow of breast milk. It contains antibodies and immunoglobulins, which help protect the newborn from bacteria and viruses and help to prevent the infant's immature gut from becoming infected. Colostrum is high in protein, zinc, and other minerals and contains less fat, carbohydrates, and calories than actual breast milk.

FACT

The size of breasts is not a factor in how much milk a mother produces. Instead it is the infant's feeding habits that control milk production. In other words, the more a woman breastfeeds her infant, the more milk her body will produce.

Between the third and sixth day after birth, colostrum begins to change to a "transitional" form of breast milk. During this time, the amounts of protein and immune factors in the milk gradually decrease while fat, lactose, and calories in the milk increase. By about the tenth day after birth, the mother begins to produce mature breast milk. One of the special qualities of breast milk is its ability to change to meet the needs of your growing baby throughout the course of breastfeeding.

The Nutrition of Breast Milk

Human breast milk provides the most optimal nutrition for infants. Breast milk seems to have the perfect balance of carbohydrates, fats, and proteins as well as vitamins and minerals that the infant needs. Breast milk contains just enough protein to keep from overloading the baby's immature kidneys. The protein in breast milk is mostly in the form of whey, which is what helps to make it easily digestible. The fat in breast milk is also easily absorbed by an infant's digestive system. Breast milk provides liberal amounts of vital essential fatty acids, saturated fats, triglycerides, and cholesterol. It contains long-chain polyunsaturated fatty acids that are essential for proper development of the central nervous system. Breast milk is relatively low in sodium and provides adequate amounts of minerals such as zinc, iron, and calcium, which reduce the demand for these nutrients from the mother.

Breast milk contains large amounts of lactose, or milk sugar. Lactose is utilized in the tissues of the brain and spinal cord and helps to provide the infant with energy. Breast milk contains only a small amount of iron, but the iron is in a form that is readily absorbed. Fifty percent of the iron in breast milk is absorbed, compared with only 4 to 10 percent of the iron in cow's milk or commercial infant formula.

The ABCs of Breastfeeding

Proper technique is important to make sure the process goes smoothly and the baby consumes enough milk. In addition to techniques, you will have plenty of questions as to how much, when, and how long. Take the time to get the advice, support, education, and encouragement you need from a lactation consultant, pediatrician, family, friends, and support groups.

ESSENTIAL

Breastfeeding requires much commitment from the mother. If you choose to go back to work outside of the home or if you are separated from your infant for other reasons, you can still breastfeed. In these cases, a breast pump can be used to collect breast milk when needed.

How Often Should I Breastfeed?

If you have chosen to breastfeed, the process should begin as soon as possible after birth. Babies who are breastfed tend to feed more often than babies who are formula fed. Breastfed babies generally eat eight to twelve times per day. This is basically because breastfed babies' stomachs empty more quickly since breast milk is so easy to digest. The baby should eat until she is full, usually ten to fifteen minutes per breast. At first, most newborns want to eat every few hours, both during the day and at night. Babies generally eat on demand when they are hungry. However, to make sure your baby is eating enough in the beginning weeks, wake her up if she has not eaten in more than four hours. Look for signs from your baby that she is hungry, such as increased alertness or activity, mouthing, or rooting around the breast. Crying seems to be more of a later sign of hunger. As your baby gets older and becomes alert for longer periods of time, you can more easily settle into a routine schedule of feeding every three hours or so with fewer sessions at night. By the end of the first month, babies will generally start sleeping longer throughout the night.

Is My Baby Getting Enough Milk?

A worry for many breastfeeding moms is whether the newborn is getting enough to eat. With formulas, you are able to tell exactly how many ounces the baby has consumed, but with breastfeeding this is harder to identify. It may seem at first that the baby is hungry all the time, which makes some moms wonder if he has had enough. This is completely normal. Babies should be hungry quite often because breast milk is digested within a couple of hours after consumption. After the baby's first few days of life, he will want to nurse about eight to twelve times per day. The baby should be fed on demand, with no worry about schedules, until you have breastfeeding down pat and can begin to recognize your baby's own schedule. The baby's pediatrician will be able to tell if your baby is getting enough to eat by how much weight he gains at each visit.

There are other ways to tell if your baby is getting enough to eat. After the fifth day of birth, she should have at least six to eight wet diapers per day and three to four loose yellow stools per day. She is most likely getting enough if she is nursing at least ten to fifteen minutes on each breast. Your baby should show steady weight gain after the first week of age. Her urine should be pale yellow and not deep yellow or orange. You should find your baby wanting to eat at least every two to three hours or at least eight times per day for at least the first two to three weeks. In addition, she should have good skin color. If you become concerned about whether your baby is getting enough to eat, contact your pediatrician or lactation consultant. Babies who are not getting enough to eat can become easily dehydrated.

FACT

In general, most babies lose a little weight, 5 to 10 percent of their birth weight, in their first few days of life. They should start to gain at least 1 ounce per day by the fifth day after birth and be back to their birth weight by two weeks after birth.

Is Breast Milk Enough?

During the first six months of life, most babies who are breastfeeding will not require any additional water, juices, vitamins, iron, or formula. With sound breastfeeding practices, supplements are rarely needed because breast milk provides the infant with just about all the fluids and nutrients he needs for proper growth and development. By six months of age, it is generally recommended that babies be introduced to foods that contain iron in addition to breast milk.

While the water supply in most U.S. cities and towns contains plenty of fluoride, a mineral often found in tap water that is important for strong teeth and prevention of cavities, in certain rural areas the levels can be too low. Breast milk contains very low levels of fluoride. However, babies under six months of age should not be given fluoride supplements, even if levels in your water supply are low.

The Vitamin D Controversy

Though breast milk is a complete source of nutrition for your baby, there is some controversy surrounding the need for supplementing with vitamin D. Vitamin D is found in only small amounts in breast milk and is necessary to absorb calcium into the bones and teeth. However, the vitamin D in breast milk is in a very absorbable form and therefore is generally adequate for most infants. Babies who may be at higher risk for vitamin D deficiency include those who have little exposure to sunlight. Moderate sunlight helps to produce vitamin D in the body, and mother and babies with darker skin may have a harder time getting enough sunlight to produce vitamin D.

Mothers deficient in vitamin D also create a risk of low levels in their babies. The amount of vitamin D in breast milk is directly related to the level of vitamin D in the mother's body. If you are taking a prenatal or vitamin/mineral supplement that contains vitamin D, drinking milk, and getting moderate exposure to sunlight, your breast milk should contain optimal levels of vitamin D. The American Academy of Pediatrics recently began recommending that all infants, including those who are exclusively breastfed, have a minimum intake of 200 international units (IU) of vitamin D per day beginning in the first two months of life.

Other Concerns

Babies sometimes react to certain foods that the mother eats because they may pass through to the breast milk. After eating spicy or gassy foods, the mother may notice the baby crying or fussing as well as nursing more often. However, these symptoms may also show up in babies with colic. You will know it is a reaction to food you have eaten if the symptoms last less than twenty-four hours. Symptoms caused by colic generally occur daily and often last for days or weeks at a time. If your baby seems to react to certain foods that you eat, eliminate those foods from your diet. If you have a family history of allergies, including asthma, you may want to avoid foods you are allergic or sensitive to while breastfeeding.

ALERT

The American Academy of Pediatrics suggests that breastfeeding mothers of susceptible infants (with a family history of allergies) are wise to eliminate peanuts and peanut-containing foods while breastfeeding.

Although the reaction is rare, some babies are allergic to cow's milk and foods that contain cow's milk in the mother's diet. Symptoms will usually appear a few minutes to a few hours after a breastfeeding session. They can include diarrhea, rash, fussiness, gas, runny nose, cough, or congestion. Talk to your pediatrician if your baby experiences any of these symptoms. Other foods you consume that may cause reactions in your newborn include chocolate, citrus fruits and juices, and common food allergens such as eggs, wheat, corn, fish, nuts, and soy.

Nutritional Requirements for the Breastfeeding Mom

As with pregnancy, it is vital that a mother eat a healthy, well-balanced diet to ensure that she gets all of the nutrients she needs for successful breast-feeding. The mother's diet must fulfill her own nutritional needs as well as additional needs, which increase during breastfeeding. At this time your body's first priority is milk production, and if you lack the right type of nourishment in your diet, your personal needs may not be met.

Calorie Needs

Your body's fuel supply for milk production comes from two main sources: extra calories, or energy, from foods you eat and energy stored as body fat during pregnancy. For your body to produce breast milk, it uses about 100 to 150 calories a day from fat that your body naturally stored during pregnancy. That is why breastfeeding moms often lose pregnancy weight more quickly. In addition, you need to eat about 500 extra calories per day (or 500 calories more than your maintenance calorie level) during breastfeeding. In general, consuming 500 more calories per day than before pregnancy will meet your energy needs for breast milk production.

Figuring on light to moderate activity, on average a woman needs about 2,700 calories per day. You need more calories if you are a teenager or more active. You can easily get these extra calories by eating nutritious foods from all of the food groups in the Food Guide Pyramid. The following number of servings from the Food Guide Pyramid would provide about 2,700 calories:

- Ten servings from the bread, cereal, rice, and pasta group (choose whole grains and whole-wheat products more often)
- Four servings from the vegetable group
- Four servings from the fruit group
- Three to four servings of dairy (choose nonfat or low-fat dairy products). Teens should shoot for 4 servings per day
- Two servings (or 6–7 ounces) from the meat, poultry, fish, dry beans, eggs, and nut group (choose leaner meats more often as well as occasionally choose nonmeat selections such as legumes, nuts, or seeds)
- Use fats and sweets sparingly

Women who were obese prior to pregnancy or who gained excessive weight during pregnancy may not require the full 500 extra calories per day. Your doctor can help to calculate the amount of additional calories you may need during breastfeeding.

Once breastfeeding is well established, a mother can reduce the number of excess calories modestly. This will increase the rate the body uses stored fat without an adverse impact on breast-milk production. Be cautious not to cut calories drastically during breastfeeding, which can reduce daily milk production.

The American Academy of Pediatrics recommends that you begin breastfeeding within the first thirty minutes of birth when possible. It is thought that this first nursing, prior to your baby's first deep sleep, imprints the correct nursing ability on their minds—not to mention that the first milk, colostrum, contains some wonderful antibodies to help protect your baby from illness and intestinal problems.

During the first two months postpartum, you will find that weight loss tends to be dramatic. It is best for you to limit your weight loss while nursing to about 4 pounds a month after the initial postpartum period is over. This is to help protect your milk supply.

How to Fuel Your Body

While you are breastfeeding, it is still important to remember that you are still eating for two. You need to continue the healthy diet you followed during pregnancy through breastfeeding and beyond. Not only is it important to get extra calories, but those extra calories need to come from healthy foods. Eating a healthy, well-balanced diet will ensure you are getting the carbohydrates, protein, and healthy fats you need for breastfeeding.

ALERT

Rapid weight loss and cutting calories too low can pose a danger to your baby. Since milk production requires extra calorie expenditure, even increasing your caloric level by 500 calories will allow for a safe amount of weight loss. Losing weight gradually through a healthy, well-balanced diet and regular exercise is the safest route.

Focus on fueling your body with whole-grain starches, fresh fruits and vegetables, and lean protein foods that will provide plenty of protein, calcium, and iron. Simply adding empty calories to increase your caloric intake, such as with sugary or high-fat foods, is not going to be advantageous to you or your baby. Eating a variety of foods is important because, this way, you can be sure to obtain different nutrients. Eating in moderation is the key—not too much of any one food or item.

Nutrient Needs of the Breastfeeding Mom

The process of breastfeeding is nutritionally demanding for a mother. During breastfeeding your need for many nutrients will increase even more than during pregnancy. The amount of milk you produce is not likely affected by the food you consume, unless you cut your calories drastically. However, the composition of your milk may vary with certain nutrients depending on your dietary intake.

Calcium

Though your calcium needs don't change during breastfeeding, calcium is still an important nutrient during this time. The recommended amount of 1,000 mg for women over nineteen is a must. If you come up short, your body may draw from the calcium reserves in your bones, which can put you at greater risk for osteoporosis later in life. It can also cause periodontal problems down the line. In addition to dairy foods, choose other foods high in calcium such as dark-green leafy vegetables, fish with edible bones, almonds, and fortified beverages.

B Vitamins

A few of the B vitamins deserve special mention, including vitamin B_{12}, folic acid, and vitamin B_6. The daily recommended intake for vitamin B_{12} increases slightly during breastfeeding. If you are a strict vegetarian, your breast milk might be missing adequate stores of vitamin B_{12}. Ensure your prenatal or multivitamin contains adequate amounts of vitamin B_{12}. If you are not a vegetarian, you most likely are getting enough. Folic acid, another B vitamin, is important especially if you are considering another pregnancy soon. The need for vitamin B_6 increases slightly during breastfeeding, and women often do not consume enough. Chicken, fish, and pork are great sources of this B vitamin as well as whole-grain products and legumes.

Iron

Iron requirements are lower after your baby is born and you are breastfeeding. The needs go down to 9 mg per day for adult women until you begin to menstruate again, in which case needs go back to normal (18 mg per day). If you are taking an iron supplement, it will not increase iron levels in your breast milk. Anemia in nursing moms has been associated with decreased milk supply. If you are anemic, you should speak to your doctor about a safe dosage of iron supplementation. You can often improve your condition by making changes to your diet. Including foods with absorbable iron sources and including a source of vitamin C with these foods can help to bring up your iron levels.

Zinc

Zinc requirements only increase slightly from pregnancy to breastfeeding. You lose some zinc when breastfeeding, and your diet may not always be able to compensate for the loss. If you are taking a prenatal or multivitamin, it should take care of any zinc requirements you may not be getting.

QUESTION

Should I exercise while I am breastfeeding?
It is safe to exercise at a moderate level after breastfeeding is well established. Aerobic exercise at 60 to 70 percent of your maximal heart rate seems to be safe and has no adverse effects on breastfeeding or milk production. However, strenuous exercise that results in lactic acid production may cause breast milk to taste sour to babies. This can happen up to ninety minutes after exercise, so plan breastfeeding sessions accordingly. Also keep in mind that you may need more calories and more fluids according to your level and frequency of exercise.

Supplements During Breastfeeding

Some doctors may recommend continuing your prenatal supplement through breastfeeding. You can get enough nutrients through the foods you eat if you consistently make good choices. If you come up short on your calories or nutrients, your breast milk is usually still sufficient for supporting your baby's proper growth and development. Unless you are severely malnourished, your breast milk will provide what the infant requires. However, this will be at the expense of your own nutrient reserves. Keep in mind that vitamin and mineral supplements should never be used to make up for poor eating habits.

Essential Fluids

You need to drink lots of fluids and stay well hydrated while breastfeeding. A hormone called oxytocin that is released by your body during breastfeeding tends to make you thirsty. Although fluids will not directly affect your milk supply, it is still recommended to drink at least eight to twelve glasses of water each day.

Harmful Substances

As with pregnancy, it is essential to think about all the substances you put into your body that can pass through to your breast milk and on to your baby. Many medications are safe to take during breastfeeding, but a few, including herbal products and/or supplements, can be dangerous to your infant. Always get approval from your doctor before taking any prescription or over-the-counter medications while breastfeeding. Alcohol should be avoided because it can pass through your breast milk to the baby. You would be wise to cut back on caffeine due to the fact that it can build up in a baby's system. A cup or two a day of coffee or cola is not likely to do harm, but too much can lead to problems. The guidelines for eating fish (due to mercury levels) also pertain to women who are breastfeeding. Habits such as smoking and illegal drugs can cause a mother to produce less milk, and chemicals such as nicotine can pass through the breast milk.

Formula Feeding

Don't beat yourself up if you cannot breastfeed for some reason. Many women cannot breastfeed for medical, physical, or other reasons. If you are not able to breastfeed or choose not to, today's infant formulas do provide a good nutritious alternative. Most are manufactured in a way that closely mimics, as much as possible, the components of breast milk. They are made to be easy for babies to digest and provide all of the nutrition needed. It is virtually impossible for a mother to create a formula at home that would have the same complex combination of proteins, sugars, fats, vitamins, and minerals that a baby needs and that are present in commercial formulas and breast milk. Therefore, if you do not breastfeed your baby, you should use only a commercially prepared formula.

What's in Formula?

Commercial formulas are usually cow-milk based and are fortified with iron as well as other essential vitamins and minerals. Some manufacturers even include some substances found directly in breast milk that can be manufactured. For infants who cannot tolerate cow's milk, there are also soy-based formulas. Formula feeding is more costly than breastfeeding but, on the other hand, is more convenient for some mothers. Today's commercial formula products are manufactured under strict sterile conditions, so there is no worry about contamination.

Because of its contents, cow's milk is not appropriate for infants younger than twelve months. Although some formulas are cow-milk based, they have been modified to meet an infant's special needs.

The Pros and Cons

Some women feel that formula-feeding their infant gives them a little more freedom and that other members of the family, such as the father, can be more active in the feeding and care of the infant. Just as breastfeeding has its own unique demands, so does formula feeding. The main demands of formula feeding are organization, handling, and proper preparation. You need to make sure to have enough formula on hand, and bottles must be prepared very carefully using sterile methods. The bottles and nipples must be kept sanitary and ready for when you need them.

Iron-fortified infant formulas have been credited for the declining incidence of iron deficiency anemia in infants. For this reason, the American Academy of Pediatrics highly recommends that mothers who are not breastfeeding use an iron-fortified infant formula.

Preparing Formulas

Commercial formulas come in all types of varieties. There are ready-to-feed liquids, concentrated liquids that require diluting with water, and powders that require mixing with water. You should always follow closely the instructions on the label for preparing bottles.

Bottle Basics

As well as varieties of formulas, there are many different types of bottles and nipples available to choose from. You may need to experiment with a few different brands before you find a combination that works best for you and your baby.

Bottles should be warmed just slightly before feeding. Never heat a bottle of formula in a microwave. The formula can heat unevenly and leave hot spots, which can burn a baby's mouth. The best way is to heat water in the microwave, take the water out, and then heat the bottle in the water. Always test the formula to make sure the temperature is not too hot. Always wash bottles and nipples thoroughly in hot water, and wash your hands before preparing them.

ALERT

Do not leave bottles out of the refrigerator for longer than one hour. If your baby doesn't finish a bottle, the contents should be discarded. If formula bottles are prepared in advance, they should be stored in the refrigerator for no longer than twenty-four hours.

How Often to Formula Feed

Experts agree that for the first few weeks, you shouldn't try to follow too rigid a feeding schedule. As the baby gets older, you may be able to work out a more established schedule. You should offer a bottle every two to three hours at first as you see signs of hunger. Until she reaches about 10 pounds, she will probably take approximately 2 to 3 ounces per feeding. From there, intake will gradually increase. Don't force her to eat if she does not seem hungry. You may see certain signs when the baby has had enough, such as closing her mouth or turning away from the bottle, falling asleep, fussiness, and biting or playing with the bottle's nipple. One advantage to bottle feeding is that you can know exactly how much your baby is eating. Your pediatrician can advise you on optimal amounts to feed your baby as she grows.

CHAPTER 20

Post-Pregnancy Nutrition

It took nine months for you to gain weight during pregnancy, so give yourself at least that much time to get your body back. Actually, giving yourself a year is more realistic if you factor in a three-month transitional period after the birth of your child. As you hammer out a routine wherein you and baby manage to get dressed and bathed before dinnertime, factor in enough time to focus on your diet and fitness routine to ensure that you're on your way to pre-baby weight in the healthiest way possible!

Post-Pregnancy Nutrition

Now that you're trying to get back into the pre-pregnancy shape, or your ideal post-pregnancy shape, it's wise to keep in mind the same healthy eating guidelines you used before and during your pregnancy and apply them to how you eat now.

Keep in mind that the type of calories you eat is also important. Those calories should come from healthy foods like fruits, vegetables, whole grains, fat-free or low-fat dairy products, lean meats, fish, poultry, and legumes. Watching your portion sizes carefully within each food group will help keep you within a moderate calorie level. Keep in mind that a gradual weight loss increases your chances of keeping the weight off. Losing weight on your own does not need to be a difficult task.

Sensible Snacking

Choosing healthy snacks is as important as the healthy meals that you plan. Healthy snacks can help you add those extra calories and nutrients you need during pregnancy as well as give you a boost of energy when you need it and take the edge off hunger in between meals. Contrary to popular belief, snacking can be part of a healthful eating plan. To keep blood sugar levels under control, it is ideal to go no longer than three or four hours between meals. The key to sensible snacking is the type and amount of food that you choose. Mindless snacking or nibbling on high-fat, high-calorie foods can lead to trouble in the form of unwanted and empty calories as well as loads of fat and sugar.

To make snacking a healthy part of your diet, choose snacks that are lower in fat and rich in nutrients. Make snacks count, instead of thinking of them as an "extra." Eat snacks well ahead of mealtime, and eat smaller portions of your snacks as opposed to big ones. Also, plan your snacks ahead of time. Good snack ideas include the following:

- Half a whole-wheat bagel or an apple topped with peanut butter
- Celery stalks with low-fat cream cheese
- Low-fat fruited yogurt topped with low-fat granola cereal
- Low-fat cottage cheese topped with fresh fruit

- Fresh fruit
- Light microwave popcorn (for extra flavor, toss with a small amount of low-fat Parmesan cheese or garlic powder)
- Pita bread stuffed with fresh veggies and low-fat ranch dressing
- Low-fat string cheese and crackers
- Raisins and rice cakes

These are only a few ideas! Use your creativity, and choose foods that you like.

QUESTION

Can eating more than three times a day be part of a healthy diet?
Yes. For women who are pregnant, nursing, or new moms who enjoy a healthy lifestyle, eating several small meals during the day can fit nicely into a healthy eating pattern. It can help you to fit in necessary calories and food group servings without having to eat large meals all at once, which can be difficult for women who may be too busy to sit down for more than just a few minutes.

Portion Power

Portion sizes are very important when you're trying to eat a healthy diet and control your calorie intake. The portion sizes you consume contribute directly to the number of calories and the amount of fat and other nutrients that you consume per day. Don't forget that even though you need a few more calories while pregnant, you are still not eating for two adult people. You can eat healthily and still be eating too much. To follow the guidelines of the Food Guide Pyramid correctly, you must be aware of the portion sizes that you eat.

Visualize Your Portions

To follow a healthy diet, you don't need to necessarily weigh and measure all of your food each day. But you do need a general idea of how much you should be eating. Keep in mind that portion sizes are meant as general guidelines—the goal is to come close to the recommended serving sizes on average over several days. Be careful of letting your stomach do the portioning. Skipping meals can lead to ravenous hunger at the next meal, which makes it difficult to correctly portion your foods. To help estimate your portion sizes, use these visual comparisons:

- A 3-ounce portion of cooked meat or poultry is about the size of a deck of playing cards.
- A medium potato is about the size of a computer mouse.
- 1 cup of rice or pasta is about the size of a fist or a tennis ball.
- An average bagel should be the size of a hockey puck or a large to-go coffee lid.
- A cup of fruit or a medium apple or orange is the size of a baseball.
- ½ cup of chopped vegetables is about the size of three regular ice cubes.
- 3 ounces of grilled fish is the size of your checkbook.
- 1 ounce of cheese is the size of four dice.
- 1 teaspoon of peanut butter equals one dice, and 2 tablespoons is about the size of a golf ball.
- 1 ounce of snack foods—such as pretzels—equals a large handful.
- A thumb tip equals 1 teaspoon, three thumb tips equal 1 tablespoon and a whole thumb equals 1 ounce.

To help you eat only the portions you measure out, portion out your food before bringing it to the table. You will be less likely to eat too much when serving bowls are not on the table. Another clever trick is to use a smaller plate to make your portion sizes look bigger.

Plan Ahead for Diet Success

There are many benefits to planning ahead that can help both your nutritional intake as well as your new (and very busy!) lifestyle. Dinner can be a much less hectic event when you know what the menu will be in advance. By planning ahead, you can make meal preparation less time-consuming, and your family will probably tend to eat together more frequently. Planning ahead also sends you to the grocery store with a list, which can help you to avoid impulse purchases (and thus save you some money!). When you plan meals, you don't tend to eat out or order out as much, which can be costly to both your pocketbook and your daily food intake.

Steps to Easy Meal Planning

Menu planning does not have to be a complicated task. A small investment of your time can reap great rewards. Menu plans can save you money by cutting out the need for last-minute trips to the grocery store. Most important, planning ahead helps conserve your most valuable resource: your energy. You don't need to plan for the next month; just plan for the next week. Keep staple foods on hand for healthy breakfasts and snacks, and then decide on a few lunches that you can eat a few times during the week. That leaves you with just seven simple dinners to plan.

Think of dishes that can be used for leftovers the next night—for instance, a pan of lasagna is sure to last you a few nights. Do your meal planning on the days that your local grocery store ads come out; this can help give you ideas for dinners for the week and will let you know which foods are on special. To come up with some ideas of meals to prepare, get out your favorite recipes or cookbooks, and see what you already have on hand. Plan meals according to your and your family's schedule, for instance, by saving the roast for a lazy Sunday and preparing a homemade pizza on the day when the kids have soccer and you work late.

Mastering Low-Fat Cooking

While planning your meals, think healthy. The methods that you use to prepare your meals can make a big difference in the amount of calories, total fat, saturated fat, and cholesterol they contain. With a few simple changes and tips to cooking methods, you can cook "leaner" and still have great-tasting dishes. Use cooking methods that require little fat, such as braising, broiling, grilling, pan-broiling, poaching, roasting, simmering, steaming, stewing, and stir-frying. Simply trimming visible fat and skin from poultry before cooking can cut fat significantly. If you leave the skin on while cooking, remove it before eating.

Other tips include running ground meat in hot water after browning and then draining to rinse off excess fat. You can also pat the meat with a paper towel or drain on a paper towel to remove excess fat. For meat that has little to no fat, try using marinades such as teriyaki sauce, orange juice, lime juice, lemon juice, tomato juice, defatted broth, or low-fat yogurt. Add fresh herbs and other spices, such as garlic powder, to marinades for more flavors. Did you ever notice that fat collects on top of stew, soups, chili, or other casserole dishes? Chill these dishes overnight and the fat will rise to the top, making it easy for you to skim off.

FACT

Grilling can be a great low-fat cooking method, but it does have a possible danger. Recent research has indicated that potential carcinogens (cancer-causing substances) may be present in grilled foods. To make grilled food safer, do not char meats or vegetables, use a low to medium heat, reduce time on the grill by baking or microwaving foods first, and avoid eating the blackened parts of grilled foods.

If you are not afraid to experiment, use half meat and half tofu, tempeh, or legumes to lower the fat in recipes and increase fiber. Stock your kitchen with nonstick saucepans, skillets, and baking pans so you can sauté and bake without adding additional fat. If you need to, use a nonstick cooking spray along with defatted broth, water, juice, or cooking wine to replace cooking oil and prevent sticking.

Healthy Up Your Recipes

In addition to using healthier cooking techniques, swapping ingredients in your recipes for leaner ones can healthy up your meals. Small changes within a recipe can make a big difference in the nutritional outcome. You may need to use less of an ingredient, substitute an ingredient, add a new ingredient, or completely leave something out. It will take some trial and error to get your recipes to your liking, but the extra effort will be well worth it.

Take a look at your recipes before you get started, and think about what individual ingredients may contribute to a dish that's higher in fat, cholesterol, calories, or sodium. Decide which ingredients can be substituted or reduced as well as added for additional nutritional value. Adding shredded carrots or zucchini to your lasagna, for example, can add a load of extra vitamins, minerals, and fiber to your dish. Make changes to your recipes gradually by changing one or two ingredients at a time each time you make it.

Use some of these substitutions to cut fat and calories while cooking or baking:

- Use fat-free or low-fat milk instead of whole milk.
- Use low-fat yogurt, ½ cup cottage cheese blended with 1½ teaspoon lemon juice, or light or fat-free sour cream instead of regular sour cream.
- Use evaporated fat-free milk or fat-free half-and-half instead of cream.
- Use 3 tablespoons cocoa powder plus 1 tablespoon vegetable or canola oil instead of 1 ounce unsweetened baking chocolate.
- Use low-fat cottage cheese or low-fat or nonfat ricotta cheese instead of regular ricotta cheese.
- Use chocolate sauce instead of fudge sauce.
- Use nonfat or low-fat plain yogurt or reduced-fat mayonnaise instead of regular mayonnaise.
- Use puréed fruits such as applesauce to replace anywhere from a third to half of the fat in recipes.
- For pies and other desserts, use a graham-cracker crumb crust instead of a higher-fat pastry shell.
- Use puréed cooked vegetables instead of cream, egg yolks, or roux to thicken sauces and soups.

Dining Out

It is nice to get out of the kitchen once in awhile and let someone else do the cooking. About half of all adults eat at a restaurant on a typical day, and almost 54 billion meals are eaten in restaurants, at school, and at work cafeterias each year. But dining out can present challenges to your goal of eating healthfully after your pregnancy.

The more meals that are eaten away from home, the bigger impact they have on your total daily nutritional intake. It is much easier to splurge or lose sight of your overall eating pattern when you eat out frequently. All of this eating out generates nutritional challenges that include larger-than-normal portion sizes, too many calories, too much fat and sodium, too few vitamins and minerals, and too little fiber.

Your Dining-Out Guidelines

Even though dining out can present some challenges, this doesn't mean you can't eat out occasionally. It simply means that you have to put some thought into the choices that you make when dining out. It also means that you will have to make a greater effort to balance out the rest of your day's intake. When you are at a restaurant, be the first to order your meal so you are not tempted by what other people order. Make an effort to eat slowly and stop eating before you feel too stuffed. You can ask the server to remove your plate once you feel full. If there is food left on your plate, ask for a doggie bag. Try splitting a meal with a dining companion, or bring half your meal home in a doggie bag for lunch the next day. In fact, you can even ask for a doggie bag to come with your meal so you can pack half of it away and not be tempted to eat the whole thing.

ESSENTIAL

Menu terms that are clues to lower-fat foods include the following words: baked, braised, broiled, grilled, roasted, steamed, stir-fried, poached, or cooked in its own juices. Menu clues that a food is likely to be higher in fat include these: Alfredo, au gratin, cheese sauce, battered, fried, béarnaise, buttered, creamed, French fried, hollandaise, pan fried, sautéed, scalloped, with gravy, or with sauce.

Start with easy changes, like choosing low-calorie salad dressings. You can also ask for dressing, gravies, sauces, and condiments (like mayonnaise) to be served on the side. This way, you have more control over how much you use. Small changes can go a long way. Don't be afraid to ask exactly how foods are prepared or to ask to have them prepared in a certain way. When choosing entrées, opt for plain meats and vegetables instead of breaded and/or deep-fried dishes, and avoid sauces and ingredients such as hollandaise, butter, cheese, and cream that can add extra calories and fat.

Request substitutes for higher-fat side dishes. For example, if your meal comes with French fries, ask for a baked potato with salsa, a brothy soup, side salad, or fresh fruit bowl instead. Be careful of appetizers before your meal that can really add up in fat and calories. Instead, choose fresh fruit, vegetable juice, marinated vegetables, raw vegetables with salsa dip, or seafood cocktail. Be very careful of beverages such as alcohol and soft drinks that can add tons of empty calories to your meal. You best bet is water with a twist of lemon—and keep it coming, especially if you're trying to avoid the bread basket! Most importantly, balance your dining-out habits with physical activity. Being physically active is what helps burn those calories. After you get home from eating out, take a walk.

Plan Ahead to Avoid Dining-Out Disasters

Planning ahead for a meal out can put you on the right path to a healthier eating experience. Plan your day so that you can fit the restaurant meal into your whole day's eating plan. Nutritional intake is what you take in over the course of an entire day, not just one meal. Never skip meals during the day just to "save up" for your night out. If you arrive at the restaurant ravenous, you will probably eat more than you intended to, and you will probably have a harder time making healthier choices. Instead, eat light meals throughout the day, and have a snack such as yogurt or fruit in the late afternoon.

Choosing a restaurant that prepares foods to order will help give you more control of what you eat and will make it easier to make special requests. This means passing up the all-you-can-eat buffets. Do some homework, and call ahead to a restaurant you plan to visit to ask about the menu and how food is prepared.

Suggestions for the Salad Bar

The salad bar always seems like a safe bet, but be aware that it can be a pitfall of excessive calories and fat if you are not careful. Choosing a large variety of vegetables and fruits can add to your day's intake of essential vitamins, minerals, and fiber. However, depending on what foods you choose, your salad bar plate can still add up to 1,000 calories or more. Excessive calories at the salad bar usually come from regular salad dressings, cheese, bacon bits, croutons, nuts or seeds, olives, and other side dishes such as macaroni salad, pasta salad, creamy soups, and even desserts.

ALERT

An order of twelve buffalo wings can weigh in at up to 700 calories and 48 grams of fat. An order of eight stuffed potato skins with sour cream can add up to 1,260 calories and 95 grams of fat. A fried onion bloom (serving size of 3 cups) with dipping sauce can add up to 2,130 calories and 163 grams of fat. Plan on skipping the appetizer and just going straight to the healthy meal.

Fumbling for Fast Food

How many times have you been out running around—or home but not in the mood to do any cooking—and decided to stop at the first fast-food place you saw? Fast foods are more popular than ever before, and many now offer a variety of healthy menu alternatives. Still, frequenting fast-food places can lead to a higher intake of fat, calories, sodium, saturated fat, and cholesterol. It can also cut into your chances of getting in all the food groups you need each day, including fruits, vegetables, dairy, and whole grains.

ALERT

We're a country of people who love our French fries. But don't be fooled into thinking this is a health food now that fast-food restaurants are telling us their fries are fried in vegetable oil. These oils are hydrogenated to make them more solid at room temperature, which means they are loaded with saturated fat.

When choosing your fast-food entrée, choose smaller burgers without the cheese, bacon, mayonnaise, and special sauces. All these toppers add more saturated fat and cholesterol to your meal, not to mention calories.

Use lower-fat toppings such as ketchup, mustard, barbecue sauces, lettuce, tomatoes, and pickles. Better yet, go for the grilled chicken breast or a sensible salad. If you choose to eat chicken or fish, stay away from the deep-fried versions, which will be high in fat and calories. A grilled, roasted, or broiled piece of chicken or fish is the healthiest choice.

Toppings can add up quickly, as follows:

- One packet of mayonnaise can have as much as 95 calories and 10 grams of fat.
- One packet of tartar sauce can add as much as 160 calories and 17 grams of fat to your fish sandwich.
- A 2-ounce packet of ranch dressing can have as much as 290 calories and 30 grams of fat.
- Just one slice of American cheese can add 50 calories and 5 grams of fat.

Subs can make for a healthy, low-fat sandwich when prepared on whole-grain bread and topped with mustard, vegetable oil, and/or low-fat cheese. Go for the cooked turkey or chicken breast instead of the higher-fat processed meats such as salami or bologna. Load up your sub with vegetables such as lettuce, tomato, onions, and peppers. Wraps are also a good choice. These are usually made from pita bread or flour tortillas and stuffed with chicken, beans, and/or vegetables. Again, beware of the added cheese, dressings, and sauces that can turn a simple sub into a high-fat and high-calorie nightmare. Ask for half the cheese, and ask for the dressing and sauce on the side so you can choose a lower-fat or fat-free version.

Not sure how your favorite fast-food menus rate? Most fast-food restaurants have websites that post nutritional information on their foods. Check them out before you head off to the drive-through!

CHAPTER 21

Getting Moving Again

Your doctor should be the one to give you the go-ahead to start slimming down or to return to exercising after delivery. This time-frame will depend on many factors, such as whether you had a vaginal or cesarean delivery, whether you experienced any complications during pregnancy such as preeclampsia or gestational diabetes, and whether you were in good shape before and during your pregnancy.

Every Body Is Different

If you were someone who was extremely fit prior to getting pregnant and you maintained a great level of fitness prior to birth, you may be ready to exercise before your other postpartum counterparts. This is also true even if you had a cesarean section. A body that was well nourished and fit will recover faster, even from major surgery. When it comes down to it, your lifestyle is one of the most important factors in your readiness to begin a new fitness program after you give birth.

For some women, pregnancy leads to permanent changes in body shape, including a more voluptuous body type with slightly wider hips and/or waistline. A majority of women lose a significant portion of the weight they gained during pregnancy within the first month of delivery. It can take up to a year to lose the remaining weight and get back your muscle tone. Of course, all women differ. This time-frame depends on many factors, including your pre-pregnancy weight and fitness level, your determination to lose the weight, your age, and your lifestyle.

Exercise and Breastfeeding

Breastfeeding is a great start not only for your baby but for you as well. You are perfectly able to nurse and exercise. In fact, nursing moms are more likely to lose their pregnancy weight than those who do not nurse.

During pregnancy, part of the fat stores your body accumulates is in preparation for nursing. These fat stores are not called upon until after the baby is born and lactation begins. You may find, as some mothers do, that these stores are not tapped into right away. They are a protective mechanism by your body to protect your baby's food supply should you find yourself in a situation where you are starving. However, these fat stores are best removed by breastfeeding.

The First Exercises After Birth

Believe it or not, the best time to begin exercise is immediately after birth. As soon as you remember, begin to think about doing exercises. You have just completed a marathon, and while you do need rest, there are certain exercises that can help you heal.

Kegels

The pelvic floor exercises that were so important before giving birth are even more important now. Remember, these perineal exercises will help increase the blood flow to that area, which will help speed the healing process and relieve pain.

At first you may have trouble isolating the muscles. This is common and you should not worry. Even if you required no stitches or sutures, the area still has been stretched to allow your baby to be born. If you did require stitches, whether or not an episiotomy was performed, you can still safely do these exercises.

Begin by doing simple flicks. You do not need to hold the counts. Merely tightening and releasing will be helpful to your recovery. You can gradually increase what you do as you feel comfortable.

Pain in this area will begin to subside and gradually get better each day. If you had stitches, they generally dissolve and do not require any special care. By the end of six weeks, your bottom should be feeling as good as new. If it isn't, be sure to talk to your doctor or midwife at your six-week checkup.

Abdominal Tightening

Abdominal tightening is a very simple exercise. It offers you the benefit of beginning to heal the abdominal muscles. It also provides you with more awareness of this area. The sooner you begin working on this, the sooner your abdomen heals and returns close to its original state.

Abdominal tightening is done simply by thinking about sucking in your abdomen. Think of pulling your belly button all the way back to your spine. Do this as you inhale. Hold the "stretch" for a few seconds, and then slowly exhale. You can do five to ten repetitions of this exercise whenever you think about it. This encourages stretched muscle fibers to shorten.

Breathing

It sounds simple, right? This time breathing has a different focus—healing. Each deep breath you take not only helps reinflate your lungs and oxygenate your body, but it enables you to heal and recover by preventing some complications of postpartum.

Resuming Exercise

Resuming exercise has many benefits. And yet society sends you mixed signals about what you should do and how you should act as a new mother. You might feel torn between resting and recuperating with baby and hurrying up and getting back to your "old self." Don't let these societal mixed messages push you.

It is important that you begin to pace yourself. Work on your fitness level and body awareness at your own speed. There are many factors that will go into your readiness to exercise.

How you gave birth will have a significant impact on when you can resume exercising regularly. While there are always simple toning exercises that can be done, many women want to know when they can get back to their normal routines. Part of the answer will depend on if you had a normal vaginal birth or a surgical birth (cesarean section).

Vaginal Birth

If you had a spontaneous vaginal birth, with or without any stitches, chances are you will be able to know when your body is ready to exercise again. For many women, this will be in fewer than the standard six weeks. There are a couple of things you will need to look for and do prior to beginning, even if you feel ready.

ESSENTIAL

If you wipe after using the bathroom and find small bits of black material on your toilet paper, do not be concerned. As the stitches reabsorb, the outside portion is sloughed off. You may notice this in your underwear, on your pad, or on the toilet paper.

The first is to see how your bleeding is doing. Typically after any birth you will bleed, called *lochia*, for up to eight weeks after the birth. This bleeding comes from your placental site and is a measure of how healed the uterus is at any given point. This bleeding will change in color and volume as you get further away from the birth. If your bleeding has stopped, you may be ready to exercise.

You need to feel well nourished and well hydrated before beginning any exercise program. These can be some of the most important signs. If you feel that all of this is in order, call your practitioner. Even if you have an appointment at the six-week postpartum mark, feel free to call earlier. Explain to the doctor or midwife that you feel your body has healed well. Tell them the status of your bleeding and your general feeling. Talk to them about starting slowly and ask what signs or symptoms you should look for, so that you would know when to cease your new routine.

Cesarean Birth

A surgical or cesarean birth is a birth, but you must also remember that it is major abdominal surgery. This alone will increase your healing time.

FACT

> The International Cesarean Awareness Network (*www.ican-online.org*) is a network designed to help women recovering from cesarean section. It can provide you with physical, mental, and emotional support after a surgical birth. There are many local chapters and peer counselors that can also help answer questions about getting your body back after abdominal surgery.

You will still bleed, just as you would with a vaginal birth. This is because the bleeding does not come from the incision but rather the placental site healing. Your iron stores and energy in general are likely to be low after surgery. A proper diet and good nutritional intake are key to healing. You may be prescribed a certain diet or vitamins to help speed this area of healing. Eating dark leafy greens, red meats, and proteins can help you fight off low iron or anemia. This can also help you feel like you have more strength.

Your practitioner will be able to help you determine when you should exercise. Since you have had surgery, this may be later than other women you know who did not. Or you may simply have to go more slowly, which is never a bad idea anyway.

Develop a Healthy Plan

Your postpartum plan is probably something you started thinking about before your pregnancy was through. While it is always great to have some vision of where you are going and where you want to be, you may find that the reality of being a new mom is more than you bargained for. Remember always to be flexible and keep in mind that your health is a top priority when trying to find your way.

ESSENTIAL

Learning to deal with change is never easy. Knowing what to expect from your body can help make this adjustment a bit easier. Realizing that you must have realistic expectations will be helpful in the road to recovery.

Once you have the physical permission and the lifestyle adjustments necessary to exercise, it is time to figure out the practicality of it all—the how, what, where, when, and whys are what really matter. It is also important to realize that the answers to these questions may change as you adapt to your new life and new roles. You should also expect to adapt nearly everything you are doing, which is where that flexibility comes in handy.

How to Exercise?

What you did prior to giving birth may be fine. You might start there with a reduced workout and slowly build it back up to where you were prior to giving birth. Then you can go forward and expand upon that base. Maybe you sense it is time for change. There are many programs designed for new mothers; in fact, there are probably more for new mothers than there are for expectant mothers.

Where to Exercise?

Where you exercise will depend on what exercises you choose. You might exercise at home in the living room while watching a taped class. Maybe you will walk around the neighborhood with some friends. Consider joining a walking club at a local mall or even a team that is taking people on to train for short runs like a 5K. You also have the option of going to a gym or other organized sporting arena.

When to Exercise?

When to exercise is always a huge question. Try not to let your new little one add to that problem. Many new moms take classes with their babies, like the stroller aerobics or other classes. You might find that your husband is more than willing to watch junior for an hour when he comes home while you walk or do an aerobics class. If you've gone back to work, consider using your lunchtime for a quick trot around the block. Or even better maybe you could bike, jog, or walk to work. Always make time to exercise.

Sample Exercise Program

Here is a sample of some of the exercises that you can safely use during the postpartum period. There are more that you can do as well, but these should be familiar to you as they are from your pregnancy exercises. Slowly move them around and add new ones as you feel able to try them. Once approved for exercise, you can also start focusing on increasing your heart rate and you don't have to worry as much about overheating as you did while you were pregnant.

Neck Stretch

Stand with your feet shoulder-width apart. Hold your shoulders up and back. The crown of your head should be pulling upward. Slowly let your chin drop to your chest and hold it there for five to ten seconds. Return your head to the neutral position. Slowly let your left ear rest on your left shoulder, again holding it for five to ten seconds. Repeat this with your right side. It is okay if you can't hold your head all the way down. Move until you feel the stretch, but without pain. Do this series three to five times.

Chest Stretch

Stand with your feet about shoulder-width apart, pelvis tucked in, and abdominals held tightly. Spread your arms to each side, at shoulder level.

Slowly curl your back forward, while bringing your arms forward as well. Allow your head to go forward slowly with this motion but try to keep the tension from your neck. As you return to a standing pose, spread your arms back to your side and feel the stretch in your chest. To ensure you feel this stretch, pull your shoulder blades together behind your back. Repeat this ten times.

Bridge on Ball

While sitting on an exercise ball, slowly walk your feet in front of you until the ball is between your shoulder blades. Keep your ankles in line with your knees and be careful not to extend your knees farther than your toes. Keep your feet as wide apart as needed to maintain your balance. When you achieve this balance, squeeze your abdominal muscles, gluteal muscles, and hamstrings as you breathe and hold the position for three to five breaths. Lower your hips after you've achieved that number of breaths, then assume the position again. Repeat it ten times.

The Figure Eight

Sitting upright on your ball, place your hands on your hips. Imagine what a figure eight looks like. Begin your figure eight, leading with the left hip, going to the right, and backward diagonally, still with your left hip. Then switch to lead with your right hip, up and back until your figure eight is completed.

Wall Pushups

Facing the wall, place your hands palm down on the wall; walk your feet backward, away from the wall. Slowly bend your elbows, bringing your upper body closer to the wall. Do about ten repetitions of the exercise. Remember to keep your spine in the proper alignment while doing this exercise.

Posture Retraining

Place your back against the wall; slowly walk your feet forward until they are 6 to 8 inches in front of you. Press your glutes, shoulder blades, and the back of your head into the wall. Slowly raise your arms at a 90-degree angle, bent elbow to the wall, and press them to the wall as well. Slowly raise your arms, keeping them on the wall, above your head.

Knee Bends

Stand with your feet slightly greater than shoulder-width apart. Begin by tilting your pelvis and begin to bend your knees. Keep your head remaining upright and don't move your feet on the floor. Return to your original pose. This is a slow motion. Do not jerk or bounce. Repeat this exercise for a total of ten repetitions.

Knee Raises

Stand with your feet slightly greater than shoulder-width apart, placing your hands on your hips or at your sides. While maintaining your proper posture, lift your right knee until it is at about a 90-degree angle. Slowly lower your leg. Repeat this exercise for a total of ten repetitions and then switch knees for another ten repetitions. For variety, alternate legs for a total of ten repetitions on each leg.

Seated Row

Sitting on the floor with a flex band wrapped around your feet at the middle of the band, hold one end of the band in each hand. Your palms should be facing the floor. Pull the band ends to your chest. Hold this for one count. Slowly release the tension in the band, returning to the original pose. Repeat this rowing motion ten times.

Cat Balance

While kneeling on the floor, pull in your abdominal muscles and breathe naturally. As you exhale, extend your right leg and left arm. Think about extending each limb as far as you comfortably can. Hold this pose for three to five breaths. Repeat ten times on each side.

Hip Abduction

Lie down on your back with your knees bent, feet flat on the floor, and your shoulders and hips firmly on the floor. Place your right ankle on your left knee. Bring your left knee toward your chest by grabbing your left thigh with your left hand. Hold this for about five seconds. Repeat on the opposite side.

Neck Roll-Ups

Lie on the floor on your back as flat as you can. Tilt your pelvis up, so that your spine is flat on the floor. Slowly begin to curl your body up from the chin to the neck, bringing your head with your chin. Pull up until your shoulder blades are off the floor. Hold this pose for five to ten seconds. Repeat ten times.

Extra Care for a Cesarean Recovery

Even if you had a normal, uneventful pregnancy, your chance of having a cesarean is nearly one in four. Since 25 percent of women will have a cesarean in the United States, you need to be aware of your risks.

The exercises for a vaginal birth are also applicable to cesarean recovery. The focus on your breathing will be stressed, because after surgery there are some complications that you are more likely to experience, like blood clots and breathing difficulties. Breathing deeply can help prevent these.

It is also imperative that you begin walking as soon as you are able to. Your intestines will be sluggish after surgery, and walking will help increase the movement of your intestines, peristalsis, as well as decrease the time of your recovery. It also helps avoid some complications of postpartum.

ESSENTIAL

Getting up for the first time after a cesarean surgery is not fun. Find a pillow or other soft object to clutch to your abdomen. You may feel like you are going to burst or that your organs will fall out. This is normal and will pass quickly, particularly the more you get up and get moving.

After a cesarean, you will also want to limit how much weight you lift or carry. A good rule is to carry nothing heavier than your baby for a few weeks. You will also want to minimize the amount of stair climbing you do. Set up a makeshift nursery downstairs. This prevents you from being isolated in your room and yet also keeps you from taking forty treks upstairs for diapers.

The First Few Days After Surgery

Having a surgical birth can leave you physically exhausted and in pain. Keep in mind that you are not only experiencing the normal postpartum occurrences, such as changes in hormones and bleeding, but you are also recovering from major abdominal surgery.

The exercises for the first few days after surgery really focus on prevention of complications. Learning to breathe after an abdominal incision is not as easy as it sounds. However, the more deep breathing you do, the less likely you are to have complications. As you hold your incision with your hands or brace it with a pillow, inhale. Put enough pressure or support on your abdomen so that you don't feel your incision will open. Do this frequently in the first few days to help prevent problems with your recovery.

In addition, try these exercises:

Walking

The first few times you get up to walk after surgery are likely to be slow and painful. Use a pillow or your hands to brace your incision. While it may feel like your organs are going to fall out, you have many layers of stitches inside your body, as well as external stitches or staples. It doesn't sound like a lot of fun, but getting up and walking will speed your recovery. The first day or two you will need someone to help you. By the second postpartum day you will probably be asked to walk around the postpartum floor or nurses' station several times a day.

Abdominal Tightening

As you lie in bed, or on the floor, have your knees bent and your feet flat on the floor. Tighten your buttocks and press your lower back into the bed or floor. As you inhale, imagine pulling your stomach down through your back to the floor or bed. Hold for up to five seconds. You can repeat this up to ten times.

Leg Slides

Lie down on your back, and bend your right leg up, leaving your left leg flat on the bed, toes up. Slide your right leg down to rest next to your left leg. Slide it back up to the bent position again. Repeat this exercise five to ten times. Then repeat it with your left leg. If you're more comfortable, try holding a pillow over your incision while you do this exercise.

The Second Week After Surgery

As your recovery progresses you will be able to do more and more. Do keep in mind that you have had major abdominal surgery, in addition to the joys of postpartum and new motherhood. Be sure to ask for help around the house and remember to allow others to do what they can. The less you do now, the faster you will heal completely.

These more advanced exercises can be tried in the second week postpartum:

Pelvic Roll

Lie on your back with your feet together. Your knees should be bent. As you hold your knees together, bring them up toward your chest. Roll them to your right side. Slowly roll them to your left side. This is a gentle rocking motion. You should avoid any jerking or bouncing while doing this. If this exercise pulls on your incision, stop doing it immediately. Repeat this up to ten times on each side.

Abdominal Strengthening

Lie down on your back with your feet together and knees slightly bent. Crisscross your arms over your abdomen, grabbing your waist on the opposite side.

As you lift your head, pull your arms together, thus pulling your stomach muscles toward each other. Try to imagine that you have an apple under your chin to ensure proper head alignment during this exercise. Don't go too far up; your shoulders should barely leave the ground when doing this. Hold the pose for three to five seconds and then relax your head and arms to the original starting position. Repeat this exercise up to five times.

The Third Week After Surgery

By now you probably feel much better, though you still have some lingering pain and tension. Be sure to listen to your body and watch your incision. Add exercises slowly to the previous week's exercises as you build your body back up:

Pelvic Tilt

After about two weeks, you can begin to do your pelvic tilts. Assume an all-fours position, on your hands and knees. Think of holding your back in its natural alignment. Then tuck only your pelvis in, bringing your pubic bone toward your neck. Be sure to move only your pelvis. If it helps, have someone hold your pelvis so that you can learn to isolate this area. Later this exercise can be done in different positions. You need to do two sets of up to ten repetitions of the pelvic tilts. Later, you can add more to each set of repetitions.

After the beginning exercises of breathing and abdominal tightening of the first few days, you will slowly begin to feel better. Your recovery will usually not be as fast as that of your vaginal-birth counterparts, but you can affect the length of time you take to recover by not doing too much.

Once you've been given the go-ahead for exercising, you will want to pay particular attention to your abdominal muscles. If you had a low transverse or bikini incision, you will not have as severe of an abdominal problem than if you required a classical or vertical incision.

Goal Setting: Now and Then

It is important to establish both short-term and long-term goals as part of your weight-loss plan. Short-term goals help you reach long-term goals by acting as small steps and keeping you motivated throughout the process. Short-term goals can help change behaviors and keep you motivated. Your goals should deal with specific problems, such as the need to eat more vegetables, and should be specific about the what, where, when, and how of your planned changes. In other words, get yourself an action plan.

Short-term goals, such as drinking 64 ounces of water each day, can help change behaviors. Be specific about how you will reach your goal. It is too vague to simply say, "I will drink more water." This does not give you any specific action to work on. On the other hand, the statement, "I will buy a 32-ounce water bottle and fill it up and drink it twice a day" is specific enough that you can measure each day whether you have achieved your goal.

Short-term goals, such as a class reunion, can also help motivate you through your weight-loss process, but make sure you line up another goal as soon as that event is over to keep you going. A specific event should not be your final or long-term goal. Make your long-term goals more than just weight loss. Make them goals that will emerge from the weight loss, such as getting healthy, defining a positive self-image, taking better care of your children, having more energy, improving the quality of your life, eating better, and enjoying physical activity.

One Step at a Time

Work on a few behaviors at a time, and once you have accomplished those, move on to a few more. Trying to bite off more than you can chew can be overwhelming as well as discouraging. Once you accomplish a short-term goal, move on to the next. A feeling of accomplishment can be a great motivational tool. Here's an example:

Long-Term Goal: Improve my health risk factors.
Short-Term Goal: Eat breakfast every day.
Action Plan: Buy healthy breakfast foods to have on hand, and get up fifteen minutes early to make time for breakfast.

APPENDIX A

Two-Week Clean Pregnancy Meal Plan

This two-week meal plan focuses on including a wide variety of natural foods throughout the day in order to satisfy the needs of mom-to-be and baby. By including a variety of fruits, vegetables, grains, and proteins in each of your day's five meals, you can maximize each meal's potential to deliver valuable nutrients and ensure your body and your baby are getting everything you need and nothing you don't. And, as always, don't forget to drink your water!

Each day of this meal plan provides an average of 1,200–1,400 calories spread evenly throughout the day's five meals and snacks. With "wiggle room" for extra calories as your unique needs would specify, the 1,200–1,400 calorie meal plan offers the opportunity for you to add other healthful foods like a handful of almonds, a cup of broccoli, an apple, etc. depending upon how your body feels on any given day throughout your pregnancy. In order to optimize your body's digestion of foods, and its use of the macro- and micronutrients they provide, you should aim to consume each meal and snack every three hours from your first meal of the day (which should be consumed within an hour of waking); for example, if you wake at 6:00 A.M., your day's meal times would be 6:30 A.M., 9:30 A.M., 12:30 P.M., 3:30 P.M., and 6:30 P.M. As a helpful hint, you could also aim to consume 8 ounces of water every hour on the hour for the first eight hours after you wake; not only can this decrease nausea symptoms, it can ensure that you stay adequately hydrated and avoid false hunger pains.

Keep in mind that each of these recipes has been chosen for the unique vitamin and mineral sources included. The iron-rich veggies, antioxidant-rich fruits, and protein-packed sources of foods you consume throughout your pregnancy should taste delicious enough that you want to eat them, and you feel satisfied choosing them over junky alternatives. Chosen with pregnancy symptoms like nausea, heartburn, and extra "pickiness" in mind, these recipes (just like those that can be found in *The Everything® Eating Clean Cookbook*) can be considered safe for most . . . and easily adaptable for others. Keep in mind that, in the event you find yourself only able to consume smoothies for a part of your pregnancy due to your pregnancy symptoms, *What Color Is Your Smoothie?* is a wonderful book packed full of over 300 smoothie recipes, each with explanations of its unique blend's healthy benefits. Asterisks signify recipes included in Appendix B.

Day 1:
- Meal/Snack #1: Strawberries, blueberries, and Greek yogurt
- Meal/Snack #2: Blazing Blueberry Muffins* (2)
- Meal/Snack #3: Tuna Salad–Stuffed Tomatoes* (2 servings)
- Meal/Snack #4: Cooked gluten-free pasta with olive oil and vegetables
- Meal/Snack #5: Pork Loin and Roasted Root Vegetables*

Day 2:
- Meal/Snack #1: Turkey, Egg-White, and Hash Brown Bake* (2 servings)
- Meal/Snack #2: Very Cherry Vanilla Smoothie*
- Meal/Snack #3: Large salad with greens, fresh vegetables, olive oil, and agave nectar
- Meal/Snack #4: Grilled Chicken and Pineapple Sandwich*
- Meal/Snack #5: Grilled lean steak with a baked potato and steamed broccoli

Day 3:
- Meal/Snack #1: Lots of Latte Smoothie*
- Meal/Snack #2: Greek yogurt with pineapple chunks, strawberry slices, and walnuts
- Meal/Snack #3: Mushroom and Asparagus Bake*
- Meal/Snack #4: Cooked, chilled tilapia with cooked peppers and onions
- Meal/Snack #5: Creamy Lemon Chicken*

Day 4:
- Meal/Snack #1: Berry Banana Smoothie*
- Meal/Snack #2: Sliced apples and bananas with Greek yogurt and agave nectar
- Meal/Snack #3: Vegetarian Meatloaf*
- Meal/Snack #4: Turkey slices, lettuce, and cranberry sauce in a whole-wheat tortilla
- Meal/Snack #5: Spinach and Mushroom Chicken*

Day 5:
- Meal/Snack #1: Fruity Egg White Frittata* (2 servings)
- Meal/Snack #2: Large spinach salad with mandarin oranges and sliced almonds
- Meal/Snack #3: Baby carrots, celery sticks, and sliced bell pepper with hummus
- Meal/Snack #4: Creamy Broccoli Soup (2 servings)*
- Meal/Snack #5: Shepherd's Pie (2 servings)*

Day 6:
- Meal/Snack #1: Smoothie made with 1 cup pineapple chunks, 1 cup coconut milk, and ice
- Meal/Snack #2: Mashed bananas, vanilla Greek yogurt, and homemade granola
- Meal/Snack #3: Tempting Tilapia and Veggie Wrap*
- Meal/Snack #4: Cabbage Rolls (2)*
- Meal/Snack #5: Grilled chicken with steamed asparagus and mashed cauliflower

Day 7:
- Meal/Snack #1: Oatmeal, baked apples, and cinnamon
- Meal/Snack #2: Pumpkin Spice Smoothie*
- Meal/Snack #3: Fruit, slivered almonds, and cottage cheese
- Meal/Snack #4: Spinach salad with raspberries, strawberries, walnuts, and agave nectar
- Meal/Snack #5: Chicken and Broccoli Fettuccine*

Day 8:
- Meal/Snack #1: 2 scrambled eggs with 1 slice sprouted grain bread
- Meal/Snack #2: Fruit Salad with Ginger and Lemon Juice*
- Meal/Snack #3: Chocolate Almond Butter Smoothie*
- Meal/Snack #4: Creamy Asparagus Soup*
- Meal/Snack #5: Grilled chicken or steak with bowtie pasta and grilled veggies

Day 9:
- Meal/Snack #1: Peaches 'n' Cream Smoothie*
- Meal/Snack #2: Almond butter and banana on a toasted whole-wheat English muffin
- Meal/Snack #3: Egg salad made with 2 hard boiled eggs, Greek yogurt, celery, and a sprinkle of salt
- Meal/Snack #4: Blackened Mahi-Mahi Sandwich*
- Meal/Snack #5: Large spinach salad with chilled cooked steak, green onions, water chestnuts, and sesame oil

Day 10:
- Meal/Snack #1: 2 slices sprouted grain bread topped with cottage cheese and maple syrup
- Meal/Snack #2: Marvelous Mediterranean Wrap*
- Meal/Snack #3: Smoothie made of water, greens (of choice), apple, banana, and ice

- Meal/Snack #4: Macaroni Salad with Sautéed Veggies and Vinaigrette*
- Meal/Snack #5: Spice-Rubbed Roasted Turkey Breast* with steamed broccolini and mashed sweet potato

Day 11:
- Meal/Snack #1: Pumpkin Flaxseed Muffins* (2)
- Meal/Snack #2: Oatmeal Berry Smoothie*
- Meal/Snack #3: Spinach salad with chopped turkey, grapes, and walnuts with Greek yogurt and agave nectar
- Meal/Snack #4: Creamy Mushroom and Rice Soup* (2 servings)
- Meal/Snack #5: Pork Loin with Baked Apples*

Day 12:
- Meal/Snack #1: Tossed fruit with cottage cheese
- Meal/Snack #2: Tasty Turkey Avocado Wrap*
- Meal/Snack #3: Very Veggie Frittata*
- Meal/Snack #4: Peeled and sliced cucumber salad with grape tomatoes, Greek yogurt, and dill
- Meal/Snack #5: Spinach-Stuffed Chicken*

Day 13:
- Meal/Snack #1: Smoothie with apples, almond milk, ground cloves, and cinnamon
- Meal/Snack #2: Cooked, chilled, shredded chicken with Greek yogurt, and sliced celery
- Meal/Snack #3: Squash Casserole*
- Meal/Snack #4: Amazing Minestrone*
- Meal/Snack #5: Roasted turkey breast, mashed sweet potatoes, and green beans

Day 14:
- Meal/Snack #1: Sweet Potato Pancakes* (2)
- Meal/Snack #2: Spinach salad topped with sliced cucumber, tomatoes, and avocado
- Meal/Snack #3: Too-Good Turkey Burger*
- Meal/Snack #4: Cherry Banana Protein Power Smoothie*
- Meal/Snack #5: Lemony Basil-Chicken* (2 servings)

APPENDIX B

Recipes

Fruity Egg White Frittata

INGREDIENTS | SERVES 6

1 cup sliced strawberries
1 cup blueberries
1 cup raspberries
10 egg whites
1 teaspoon vanilla extract
1 tablespoon agave nectar

1. Preheat oven to 350°F and spray an oven-safe frying pan with olive oil cooking spray.

2. Over medium heat, sauté all fruit together until lightly heated and softened.

3. While fruit is heating, whisk together the egg whites, vanilla, and agave nectar briskly until well blended. Add to the frying pan, covering fruit completely.

4. Continue cooking until the center solidifies slightly and bubbles begin to appear.

5. Remove from heat and place into preheated oven.

6. Cook for 10–15 minutes, or until frittata is firm in the center.

PER SERVING Calories: 70 | Fat: 0.5 g | Protein: 6.5 g | Sodium: 92 mg | Fiber: 2.5 g | Carbohydrates: 11 g | Sugar: 7.5 g

Turkey, Egg White, and Hash Brown Bake

INGREDIENTS | SERVES 16

1 pound ground turkey breast, browned
1 pound shredded potatoes
16 egg whites
4 whole eggs
2 teaspoons all-natural sea salt
2 teaspoons freshly ground black pepper
1 teaspoon cayenne pepper

1. Preheat oven to 375°F.

2. Spray a 9" × 13" glass casserole dish with olive oil cooking spray.

3. Combine ground turkey breast, potatoes, egg whites, and eggs thoroughly.

4. Season with salt, black pepper, and cayenne.

5. Pour mixture into baking dish and let settle completely.

6. Bake for 30–40 minutes, or until top is golden and firm and inserted fork comes out clean.

PER SERVING Calories: 92 | Fat: 2.6 g | Protein: 11 g | Sodium: 387 mg | Fiber: 0.5 g | Carbohydrates: 6 g | Sugar: 0.2 g

Blazing Blueberry Muffins

INGREDIENTS | SERVES 12

¾ cup 100% whole-wheat baking flour

¾ cup bran flakes cereal, crushed

½ cup Sucanat

½ teaspoon baking soda

1 teaspoon cinnamon

¼ cup unsweetened applesauce

1 cup mashed ripe bananas

½ cup vanilla almond milk

2 eggs

1 teaspoon vanilla extract

1 cup fresh blueberries

1. Preheat oven to 425°F.

2. Grease a 12-cup muffin pan or line with paper baking cups.

3. Combine flour, cereal, Sucanat, baking soda, and cinnamon in a large mixing bowl. Add applesauce, bananas, almond milk, eggs, and vanilla and mix well. Gently fold in blueberries.

4. Pour muffin mix evenly into each of the muffin cups.

5. Bake for 20 minutes, or until a fork inserted into the center of a muffin comes out clean.

PER SERVING Calories: 109 | Fat: 1.3 g | Protein: 3 g | Sodium: 35 mg | Fiber: 2.3 g | Carbohydrates: 23 g | Sugar: 12 g

Pumpkin Flaxseed Muffins

INGREDIENTS | SERVES 12

¾ cup 100% whole-wheat flour

½ cup ground flaxseed

½ cup Sucanat

½ teaspoon baking powder

1 teaspoon baking soda

1 teaspoon pumpkin pie spice

1½ cups pumpkin purée

½ cup vanilla almond milk

2 eggs

3 tablespoons agave nectar

1 teaspoon vanilla extract

1. Preheat oven to 375°F.

2. Grease a 12-cup muffin pan or line with paper baking cups.

3. Combine flour, flaxseed, Sucanat, baking powder, baking soda, and pumpkin pie spice in a large mixing bowl. Add pumpkin purée, almond milk, eggs, agave nectar, and vanilla. Blend well.

4. Pour muffin mix evenly into each of the muffin cups.

5. Bake for 20 minutes, or until a fork inserted into the center of a muffin comes out clean.

PER SERVING Calories: 138 | Fat: 4 g | Protein: 4 g | Sodium: 37 mg | Fiber: 3.3 g | Carbohydrates: 24 g | Sugar: 14 g

Sweet Potato Pancakes

INGREDIENTS | SERVES 10

1 cup sweet potato purée
1 cup plain low-fat Greek-style yogurt
1 cup unsweetened applesauce
2 egg whites
2 whole eggs
2 teaspoons vanilla
2 tablespoons Sucanat
¼ cup 100% whole-wheat flour
1 teaspoon baking powder
1 teaspoon pumpkin pie spice
1 teaspoon cinnamon
2 tablespoons agave nectar

1. Coat a nonstick skillet with olive oil cooking spray and place over medium heat.

2. Combine all ingredients except agave nectar and mix well.

3. Scoop the batter onto the preheated skillet, using approximately ½ cup of batter per pancake.

4. Cook 2–3 minutes on each side, or until golden brown. Remove from heat, plate, and drizzle all pancakes with the agave nectar.

PER SERVING Calories: 78 | Fat: 1 g | Protein: 7 g | Sodium: 52 mg | Fiber: 1 g | Carbohydrates: 13 g | Sugar: 6 g

Very Veggie Frittata

INGREDIENTS | SERVES 4

½ cup chopped broccoli
½ cup mushrooms, cleaned and diced
½ cup chopped yellow pepper
¼ onion, chopped finely
¼ cup filtered water
6 egg whites
6 eggs
1 tablespoon garlic powder
1 teaspoon all-natural sea salt
2 teaspoons freshly ground black pepper

1. Preheat oven to 350°F. Spray a large oven-safe skillet with olive oil cooking spray, and preheat over medium heat.

2. Combine broccoli, mushrooms, pepper, and onion in the skillet with the water and cook until tender, but not soft.

3. Whisk together egg whites, eggs, garlic powder, salt, and pepper and pour over veggie mixture.

4. Cook until the center begins to shake and bubble from the heat (about 3–4 minutes). Remove from heat and place in preheated oven for 15 minutes, or until center is set and an inserted fork comes out clean.

PER SERVING Calories: 181 | Fat: 8 g | Protein: 17 g | Sodium: 788 mg | Fiber: 4.5 g | Carbohydrates: 13 g | Sugar: 1.7 g

Berry Banana Smoothie

INGREDIENTS | SERVES 2

2 bananas, peeled

1 cup strawberries

1 cup blueberries

1 cup strawberry kefir

1 teaspoon vanilla extract

2 cups ice

1. Combine bananas, berries, kefir, and vanilla extract in the blender with 1 cup of the ice and blend until thoroughly combined.

2. Add remaining cup of ice gradually while blending until desired consistency is reached.

PER SERVING Calories: 252 | Fat: 4.5 g | Protein: 6 g | Sodium: 61 mg | Fiber: 7.5 g | Carbohydrates: 50 g | Sugar: 31 g

Very Cherry Vanilla Smoothie

INGREDIENTS | SERVES 2

2 cups cherries, pitted

1 banana, peeled

Pulp of 1 vanilla bean

1 cup vanilla almond milk

1 teaspoon vanilla extract

1 cup ice

1. Combine cherries, bananas, vanilla bean pulp, almond milk, and vanilla extract in the blender with ½ cup of the ice and blend until thoroughly combined.

2. Add remaining ½ cup of ice gradually while blending until desired consistency is reached.

PER SERVING Calories: 200 | Fat: 4.5 g | Protein: 3.5 g | Sodium: 202 mg | Fiber: 6 g | Carbohydrates: 40 g | Sugar: 27 g

Pumpkin Spice Smoothie

INGREDIENTS | SERVES 2

1 cup sweet potato purée
1 cup vanilla almond milk
1 teaspoon ground cloves
1 teaspoon ginger
1 teaspoon cinnamon
2 cups ice

1. Combine sweet potato purée, almond milk, and spices in the blender with 1 cup of the ice and blend until thoroughly combined.

2. Add remaining cup of ice gradually while blending until desired consistency is reached.

PER SERVING Calories: 118 | Fat: 4 g | Protein: 2.5 g | Sodium: 227 mg | Fiber: 3.8 g | Carbohydrates: 19 g | Sugar: 4.6 g

Peaches 'n' Cream Smoothie

INGREDIENTS | SERVES 2

2 cups fresh chopped peaches
1 banana, peeled
2 cups vanilla almond milk
2 cups ice

1. Combine peaches, banana, and almond milk in the blender with ½ cup of the ice and blend until thoroughly combined.

2. Add remaining ice gradually while blending until desired consistency is reached.

PER SERVING Calories: 202 | Fat: 8.4 g | Protein: 4.2 g | Sodium: 403 mg | Fiber: 6 g | Carbohydrates: 32 g | Sugar: 20 g

Chocolate Almond Butter Smoothie

INGREDIENTS | SERVES 2

1 banana, peeled
4 dates, pitted
¼ cup raw cocoa
½ cup natural almond butter
2 cups vanilla almond milk
2 cups ice

1. Combine the banana, dates, cocoa, almond butter, and almond milk in the blender with ½ cup of the ice and blend until thoroughly combined.

2. Add remaining ice gradually while blending until desired consistency is reached.

PER SERVING Calories: 473 | Fat: 25 g | Protein: 10.5 g | Sodium: 411 mg | Fiber: 11 g | Carbohydrates: 63 g | Sugar: 38 g

Oatmeal Berry Smoothie

INGREDIENTS | SERVES 2

1 cup blueberries

1 cup raspberries

½ cup dry rolled oats

2½ cups blueberry kefir

2 teaspoons cinnamon

2 cups ice

1. Combine berries, oats, kefir, and cinnamon in the blender with ½ cup of the ice and blend until thoroughly combined.

2. Add remaining ice gradually while blending until desired consistency is reached.

PER SERVING Calories: 345 | Fat: 11 g | Protein: 13 g | Sodium: 148 mg | Fiber: 12.5 g | Carbohydrates: 51 g | Sugar: 24 g

Cherry Banana Protein Power Smoothie

INGREDIENTS | SERVES 2

1 large banana, peeled

1 cup cherries, pitted

2 cups vanilla almond milk

1 cup ice

1. Combine banana, cherries, and almond milk in a blender with ½ cup of ice and blend until thoroughly combined.

2. Add remaining ½ cup of ice as needed while blending until desired consistency is achieved.

PER SERVING Calories: 198 | Fat: 8 g | Protein: 3.7 g | Sodium: 403 mg | Fiber: 5.6 g | Carbohydrates: 32 g | Sugar: 18 g

Lots of Latte Smoothie

INGREDIENTS | SERVES 2

2 cups prepared coffee, cooled

2 cups vanilla almond milk

2–3 cups ice

1 tablespoon agave nectar

1. Combine the coffee, almond milk, and ½ of the ice in a blender, and blend until thoroughly combined.

2. Add remaining ice while blending until desired consistency is achieved.

3. Add agave nectar gradually while blending until desired sweetness is achieved.

PER SERVING Calories: 124 | Fat: 7.8 g | Protein: 2.5 g | Sodium: 408 mg | Fiber: 2.3 g | Carbohydrates: 13 g | Sugar: 8.7 g

Tuna Salad–Stuffed Tomatoes

INGREDIENTS | SERVES 6

1 can solid white albacore tuna, packed in water

½ cup plain low-fat yogurt

¼ cup chopped celery

¼ cup finely minced onion

1 teaspoon garlic powder

1 teaspoon all-natural sea salt, or to taste

1 teaspoon freshly ground black pepper

6 Roma tomatoes, tops and seeds removed

1. In a large mixing bowl, crush the drained tuna.

2. Add ½ cup of the low-fat yogurt, celery, onion, and garlic powder. Taste and add salt and pepper as needed.

3. Fill each cleaned tomato with ⅙ of the tuna mixture.

PER SERVING Calories: 92 | Fat: 3 g | Protein: 10.6 g | Sodium: 523 mg | Fiber: 1 g | Carbohydrates: 6 g | Sugar: 4 g

Marvelous Mediterranean Wraps

INGREDIENTS | SERVES 2

½ cup sun-dried tomatoes

4 tablespoons plain low-fat Greek-style yogurt

1 grilled boneless, skinless chicken breast, torn into bite-sized pieces

½ cup roasted red peppers

½ cup sliced olives

½ cup artichoke hearts, chopped

1 teaspoon garlic powder

1 teaspoon all-natural sea salt

2 100% whole-wheat tortillas

1. Soak tomatoes in warm water for 30 minutes. Drain and pat dry.

2. In a mixing bowl, combine the yogurt, chicken, sun-dried tomatoes, red peppers, olives, artichokes, and garlic powder. Add salt to taste.

3. Lay tortillas on a flat surface and spoon half of the mixture down the center of each wrap.

4. Wrap tightly and enjoy!

PER SERVING Calories: 352 | Fat: 9 g | Protein: 33 g | Sodium: 1587 mg | Fiber: 6 g | Carbohydrates: 35 g | Sugar: 10 g

Tempting Tilapia and Veggie Wraps

INGREDIENTS | SERVES 2

1 small onion, sliced in strips
1 yellow squash, sliced
1 zucchini, sliced
2 tablespoons olive oil, divided
2 garlic cloves, crushed
1 lemon, juiced
2 100% whole-wheat tortillas
1 pound tilapia fillet
1 teaspoon all-natural sea salt
1 teaspoon freshly ground black pepper

1. Over medium heat, prepare a large skillet with olive oil spray.

2. Add onion slices, squash, and zucchini, and drizzle with 1 tablespoon of the olive oil. Sauté for 4–5 minutes, then add crushed garlic and half of the lemon juice. Continue sautéing for 5 minutes, or until all vegetables are slightly softened.

3. Remove vegetables from the heat and place equal servings in mounds on the two tortillas.

4. Return skillet to medium heat and drizzle with remaining tablespoon of olive oil.

5. Rinse tilapia fillet and place in heated skillet with the rest of the lemon juice.

6. Allow fillet to cook undisturbed for 3–5 minutes or until fish begins to whiten through.

7. Flip fillet and continue cooking for 5 minutes, or until fish is flaky and no juices remain.

8. Remove fish from heat, crumble or halve, and place atop each vegetable mound with salt and pepper to taste.

PER SERVING Calories: 453 | Fat: 18 g | Protein: 45 g | Sodium: 1000 mg | Fiber: 4 g | Carbohydrates: 28 g | Sugar: 7 g

Too-Good Turkey Burgers

INGREDIENTS | SERVES 4

½ cup chopped onions
1 pound ground turkey breast
1 teaspoon minced garlic
1 teaspoon all-natural sea salt
1 teaspoon freshly ground black pepper
4 100% whole-wheat hamburger buns
1 cup shredded romaine hearts
4 slices beefsteak tomato

1. Prepare a grill with olive oil spray and heat to medium heat.

2. Prepare a sauté pan with olive oil spray over medium heat, and add onions. Sauté until soft and translucent.

3. In a large mixing bowl, add the ground turkey breast, minced garlic, sautéed onions, salt, and pepper, and combine thoroughly. Form into 4 patties of the same size.

4. Place patties on the open grill's flame, and cook for 5–7 minutes undisturbed.

5. Flip the patties and continue cooking for 5–7 minutes, or until juices run clear.

6. Open the buns, and move each patty to the bottom half of each bun.

7. Top burgers with the sliced tomato, shredded lettuce, and bun top, and enjoy!

PER SERVING Calories: 225 | Fat: 2.5 g | Protein: 30 g | Sodium: 754 mg | Fiber: 2.8 g | Carbohydrates: 19 g | Sugar: 2.7 g

Tasty Turkey Avocado Wraps

INGREDIENTS | SERVES 2

4 slices roasted turkey breast (⅛" thick)
1 avocado, skin and seed removed
2 100% whole-wheat tortillas
2 tablespoons lemon juice
½ cup diced tomatoes
1 teaspoon chopped mint

1. Cut turkey breast slices into thin strips, separating into two equal servings.

2. Slice the avocado into thin strips.

3. Lay the tortillas flat and place each serving of the turkey breast down the center of each wrap. Lay the avocado slices over the turkey, and drizzle with the lemon juice.

4. Top the avocado with the diced tomato and mint, wrap tightly, and enjoy!

PER SERVING Calories: 358 | Fat: 18 g | Protein: 24 g | Sodium: 254 mg | Fiber: 8 g | Carbohydrates: 26 g | Sugar: 2.7 g

Grilled Chicken and Pineapple Sandwiches

INGREDIENTS | SERVES 2

2 skinless, boneless chicken breasts
½ cup freshly juiced pineapple juice
4 pineapple slices of ¼" thickness
2 100% whole-wheat buns

1. Prepare a grill with olive oil spray to medium heat.

2. Place the chicken breasts on the hot grill and pour ¼ cup of the pineapple juice over the breasts. Cook for 7 minutes.

3. Turn the breasts over, and pour the remaining pineapple juice over the breasts. Continue cooking for another 7 minutes or until juices run clear.

4. Place the pineapple slices on the grill and cook for 3 minutes before turning. Remove chicken and pineapple slices from the grill, stack on whole wheat buns, and enjoy!

PER SERVING Calories: 542 | Fat: 7 g | Protein: 54 g | Sodium: 412 mg | Fiber: 6.8 g | Carbohydrates: 65 g | Sugar: 41 g

Blackened Mahi-Mahi Sandwiches

INGREDIENTS | SERVES 2

1 teaspoon cayenne pepper

1 teaspoon paprika

1 teaspoon cumin

1 teaspoon freshly ground black pepper

1 teaspoon all-natural sea salt

1 teaspoon onion powder

2 mahi-mahi fillets (about 1 pound), rinsed

4 slices sprouted grain bread

1 cup shredded romaine hearts

2 slices beefsteak tomato

2 tablespoons plain nonfat yogurt

¼ cup freshly squeezed lime juice

1 tablespoon chopped mint

1. Prepare a large skillet over medium heat with olive oil spray.

2. Mix the cayenne, paprika, cumin, pepper, salt, and onion powder in a shallow dish and completely coat fish on both sides by dredging them in the spice mix.

3. Place the fillets on the hot skillet and cook for 4–5 minutes on each side or until crispy and flaky.

4. Place the two fillets on two separate slices of the bread, and top with the shredded lettuce and tomato.

5. In a small mixing bowl, combine the yogurt, lime juice, and mint, and spread half of the mixture on each piece of bread intended to top the sandwiches, and cover.

PER SERVING Calories: 276 | Fat: 2.3 g | Protein: 32 g | Sodium: 1140 mg | Fiber: 2 g | Carbohydrates: 5.4 g | Sugar: 1.8 g

Pork Loin and Roasted Root Vegetables

INGREDIENTS | SERVES 4

4 Idaho potatoes

4 carrots, peeled and tops removed

2 yellow onions, skin removed

2 tablespoons olive oil

2 teaspoons all-natural sea salt, divided

2 teaspoons freshly ground black pepper, divided

2 teaspoons smoked paprika, divided

1 teaspoon turmeric

1 pound pork tenderloin

1. Preheat oven to 400°F, and prepare a 9" × 13" baking dish with olive oil spray.

2. Cut potatoes, carrots, and onions in similar bite-sized pieces.

3. In a large resealable plastic bag, combine the potatoes, carrots, onions, and olive oil with 1 teaspoon of the salt, 1 teaspoon of the pepper, 1 teaspoon of the paprika, and the turmeric, and toss to coat evenly.

4. Pour the vegetables in an even layer in the prepared dish.

5. Cook at 400°F for 30 minutes.

6. Remove veggies from the oven, stir, and clear a space large enough to fit the pork tenderloin in the middle of the vegetables. Top the pork loin with the remaining spices.

7. Return the pan to the oven, and continue cooking at 400°F for 30–40 minutes, or until meat thermometer inserted in the center of the pork reads 165°F.

PER SERVING Calories: 388.29 | Fat: 9.86 g | Protein: 28.65 g | Sodium: 1304.12 mg | Fiber: 8.90 g | Carbohydrates: 47.20 g | Sugar: 8.34 g

Shepherd's Pie

INGREDIENTS | SERVES 16

2 pounds browned ground turkey breast
1 onion, minced
4 teaspoons garlic powder
4 teaspoons onion powder
2 teaspoons all-natural sea salt
2 teaspoons freshly ground black pepper
4 cups frozen peas
4 cups mashed potatoes or mashed cauliflower

1. Preheat oven to 350°F and spray a 9" × 13" dish with olive oil spray.

2. In a mixing bowl, combine the browned ground turkey breast, half of the minced onion, 2 teaspoons of the garlic powder, 2 teaspoons of the onion powder, 1 teaspoon of the salt, and 1 teaspoon of the pepper, and blend well.

3. Layer the meat on the bottom of the pan, cover with the peas, and sprinkle with the remaining minced onion.

4. Stir the remaining spices into the mashed potatoes or cauliflower, and spoon over the peas, spreading evenly.

5. Bake at 350°F for 30 minutes, or until top begins to turn golden.

PER SERVING Calories: 149.08 | Fat: 1.26 g | Protein: 17.41 g | Sodium: 461.54 mg | Fiber: 2.19 g | Carbohydrates: 16.70 g | Sugar: 2.40 g

Spinach and Mushroom Chicken

INGREDIENTS | SERVES 2

2 boneless, skinless chicken breasts
1 tablespoon olive oil
2 cups baby portabella mushrooms
2 cups baby spinach leaves
2 teaspoons garlic powder
1 teaspoon all-natural sea salt
1 teaspoon freshly ground black pepper

1. Prepare a skillet with olive oil spray over medium heat.

2. Cut chicken into 1" pieces. Pour the tablespoon of olive oil and mushrooms into the skillet and sauté for 3–4 minutes.

3. Add chicken and sauté for 5 minutes.

4. When mushrooms are softened and chicken is thoroughly cooked through, add spinach leaves and seasonings, and sauté for 1 minute or until spinach is wilted.

5. Remove from heat and serve.

PER SERVING Calories: 230.76 | Fat: 10.67 g | Protein: 27.21 g | Sodium: 1298.85 mg | Fiber: 2.31 g | Carbohydrates: 7.15 g | Sugar: 2.35 g

Chicken and Broccoli Fettuccine

INGREDIENTS | SERVES 2

2 tablespoons olive oil

1 boneless, skinless chicken breast

1 teaspoon minced garlic

1 cup broccoli florets

2 tablespoons filtered water

1½ cups cooked whole-wheat fettuccine

1 teaspoon all-natural sea salt

1. Prepare a skillet with 1 tablespoon of olive oil over medium heat.

2. Cut chicken breast into 1" pieces, and sauté for 2–3 minutes.

3. Add minced garlic, broccoli, and 1 tablespoon of water to skillet and continue sautéing for 4–5 minutes.

4. Add water as needed to prevent sticking and promote steaming.

5. Remove from heat when broccoli is slightly softened and the chicken is cooked through with juices running clear.

6. Toss the chicken and broccoli with the fettuccine and remaining tablespoon of olive oil. Season with the teaspoon of salt to taste.

PER SERVING Calories: 369.46 | Fat: 16.38 g | Protein: 19.44 g | Sodium: 1239.02 mg | Fiber: 3.10 g | Carbohydrates: 35.89 g | Sugar: 1.38 g

Spice-Rubbed Roasted Turkey Breast

INGREDIENTS | SERVES 8

1 (5-pound) turkey breast

2 teaspoons garlic powder

2 teaspoons onion powder

1 teaspoon cayenne

1 teaspoon all-natural sea salt

1 teaspoon freshly ground black pepper

1 tablespoon olive oil

1 lemon, sliced

1. Preheat oven to 325°F, and prepare a roasting pan with olive oil spray. Set the turkey breast in roasting pan (make sure it is thawed).

2. Combine all spices in a small mixing bowl, and mix well.

3. Coat the turkey breast with the olive oil, and sprinkle spice mixture over the turkey breast. Top with lemon slices.

4. Cook the turkey breast for 1½–2½ hours, or until internal temperature reads 165–170°F.

PER SERVING Calories: 331.38 | Fat: 3.57 g | Protein: 69.11 g | Sodium: 432.97 mg | Fiber: 0.28 g | Carbohydrates: 1.26 g | Sugar: 0.08 g

Creamy Lemon Chicken

INGREDIENTS | SERVES 2

2 boneless, skinless chicken breasts
½ cup freshly squeezed lemon juice
¼ cup plain Greek-style yogurt
2 teaspoons all-natural sea salt
1 teaspoon freshly ground black pepper
1 tablespoon chopped basil leaves

1. Cut chicken breasts into 1" pieces.

2. Prepare a skillet with olive oil spray over medium heat.

3. Pour lemon juice into skillet.

4. Once lemon juice begins to simmer, add the Greek-style yogurt and stir until the mixture becomes a sauce.

5. Add chicken, and simmer in sauce until chicken is cooked through and juices run clear.

6. Remove from heat and share the chicken evenly between two plates.

7. Cover chicken with lemon cream sauce, season with salt and pepper, and garnish with chopped basil.

PER SERVING Calories: 167.44 | Fat: 3.67 g | Protein: 27.64 g | Sodium: 2471.98 mg | Fiber: 0.55 g | Carbohydrates: 5.95 g | Sugar: 2.71 g

Spinach-Stuffed Chicken

INGREDIENTS | SERVES 2

2 boneless, skinless chicken breasts
¾ cup crumbled goat cheese
1 cup baby spinach leaves, measured then chopped
1 teaspoon freshly ground black pepper

1. Preheat oven to 350°F and prepare a baking sheet with aluminum foil and olive oil spray.

2. Slice a 2"–3" pocket in each chicken breast by gliding a knife through the side, leaving the top intact to hold the stuffing in place.

3. In a mixing bowl, combine the goat cheese and chopped spinach, stuff the chicken breasts with even amounts of the mixture, and close sides securely with toothpicks.

4. Season chicken breasts with pepper and cook for 25–30 minutes or until chicken is golden brown and juices run clear.

PER SERVING Calories: 519.13 | Fat: 33.43 g | Protein: 50.14 g | Sodium: 389.20 mg | Fiber: 0.61 g | Carbohydrates: 3.06 g | Sugar: 1.89 g

Pork Loin with Baked Apples

INGREDIENTS | SERVES 4

¼ cup unsweetened applesauce

2 tablespoons filtered water

3 Gala apples, cored, peeled, and cut into slices

1 teaspoon cinnamon

1 pound pork tenderloin

1 teaspoon all-natural sea salt

1 tablespoon agave nectar

1. Preheat oven to 400°F and spray a 9" × 13" pan with olive oil spray.

2. Mix applesauce, water, and apples in a mixing bowl with cinnamon.

3. Layer the apples evenly in the pan, and cook for 20 minutes, or until slightly softened.

4. Place pork tenderloin in the middle of the pan and surround with apples.

5. Sprinkle the tenderloin with the sea salt, and drizzle the agave nectar over the pork and the apples.

6. Return the pan to the oven for another 30 minutes, or until the internal temperature reads 165°F.

PER SERVING Calories: 203.95 | Fat: 2.61 g | Protein: 23.85 g | Sodium: 649.6 mg | Fiber: 2.05 g | Carbohydrates: 21.95 g | Sugar: 18.0 g

Lemony-Basil Chicken

INGREDIENTS | SERVES 2

2 boneless, skinless chicken breasts
1 lemon, juiced
1 teaspoon all-natural sea salt
1 teaspoon garlic powder
2 teaspoons Italian seasoning
4 tablespoons chopped fresh basil leaves
1 lemon, sliced

1. Preheat oven to 350°F, and prepare a 9" × 9" casserole dish with olive oil spray.

2. Place chicken breasts in the casserole dish and pour lemon juice over the breasts.

3. Sprinkle the breasts with salt, garlic powder, Italian seasoning, and basil leaves.

4. Cover the seasoned breasts with the lemon slices, and cook for 20–25 minutes, or until cooked thoroughly and juices run clear.

PER SERVING Calories: 155.95 | Fat: 3.67 g | Protein: 24.99 g | Sodium: 1267.34 mg | Fiber: 1.84 g | Carbohydrates: 6.56 g | Sugar: 1.5 g

Squash Casserole

INGREDIENTS | SERVES 6–8

1 large zucchini
1 large yellow squash
1 butternut squash
2 tablespoons olive oil
2 tablespoons Italian seasoning
1 tablespoon paprika
2 teaspoons all-natural sea salt
2 cups cooked brown rice
½ cup crumbled goat cheese

1. Cut the squashes into bite-sized pieces (strips or rounds) of comparable size.

2. Preheat the oven to 400°F and prepare a 9" × 13" baking dish with olive oil spray.

3. In a large mixing bowl, combine the squashes, olive oil, and seasonings, and mix well.

4. Fold in the rice and goat cheese, and bake for 35–45 minutes or until cooked through and bubbly.

PER SERVING Calories: 154.37 | Fat: 8.95 g | Protein: 5.83 g | Sodium: 640.69 mg | Fiber: 1.445 g | Carbohydrates: 13.01 g | Sugar: 1.01 g

Vegetarian Meatloaf

INGREDIENTS | SERVES 4

1 cup cooked brown rice

1 pound portabella mushrooms, minced and sautéed

1 small yellow onion, minced

1 red pepper, minced

1 cup spinach, chopped

1 cup wheat germ, plain

2 eggs, beaten

1 tablespoon vegetarian Worcestershire sauce

2 teaspoons garlic powder

2 teaspoons onion powder

2 teaspoons all-natural sea salt

2 teaspoons freshly ground black pepper

1. Preheat oven to 350°F and prepare a 9" × 9" baking dish with olive oil spray.

2. Combine all ingredients in a mixing dish, and refrigerate for 1 hour.

3. Pour mix into the center of the baking dish and form into a loaf.

4. Bake at 350°F for 30–45 minutes or until cooked through.

PER SERVING Calories: 251.79 | Fat: 6.24 g | Protein: 14.53 g | Sodium: 1280 mg | Fiber: 7.85 g | Carbohydrates: 38.56 g | Sugar: 5.45

Cabbage Rolls

INGREDIENTS | SERVES 12

1 tablespoon olive oil
1 red pepper, minced
1 yellow pepper, minced
½ red onion, minced
1 small zucchini, minced
3 garlic cloves, crushed and minced
12 red cabbage leaves
1 cup cooked brown rice
1 egg, beaten
1 teaspoon all-natural sea salt
1 teaspoon freshly ground black pepper
1 teaspoon Worcestershire sauce
1 cup marinara sauce

1. Prepare a large skillet with the tablespoon of olive oil over medium heat, and sauté the red pepper, yellow pepper, red onion, zucchini, and garlic until softened, about 5 minutes.

2. In a large pot, boil cabbage leaves for 2–4 minutes, or until soft.

3. In a mixing bowl, combine the rice, sautéed veggies, egg, salt, pepper, and Worcestershire sauce and blend well.

4. Put a ¼ cup mound of the mix in the center of each cabbage leaf, roll to close, and tuck the ends.

5. Prepare a slow cooker to low heat, and pour a couple of tablespoons of the sauce in the bottom to coat and prevent sticking. Place the rolls in the slow-cooker, and cover with sauce.

6. Cook for 8 hours, remove from heat, plate, and sprinkle with salt and pepper.

PER SERVING Calories: 67.32 | Fat: 1.88 g | Protein: 2.58 g | Sodium: 329.95 mg | Fiber: 3.12 g | Carbohydrates: 11.40 g | Sugar: 4.45 g

Mushroom and Asparagus Bake

INGREDIENTS | SERVES 8

2 cups chopped asparagus spears

1 cup portabella mushrooms, sliced

1 cup oyster mushrooms, sliced

1 cup cremini mushrooms, sliced

1 tablespoon olive oil

1 tablespoon filtered water

4 cups cooked 100% whole-wheat farfalle pasta

2 teaspoons garlic powder

1 teaspoon freshly ground black pepper

1 cup plain nonfat yogurt

1 cup plain Greek-style yogurt

1 cup crumbled goat cheese

1. Preheat oven to 350°F, and prepare a 9" × 13" baking dish with olive oil spray.

2. Prepare a skillet with olive oil spray over medium heat. Sauté the asparagus and mushrooms in the olive oil until slightly softened, about 4–6 minutes, adding water as needed to prevent sticking and promote steaming.

3. Remove veggies from heat and toss with the pasta in a mixing bowl. Add the seasonings, yogurts, and goat cheese, and blend thoroughly.

4. Pour the mix into the baking dish and bake for 30 minutes, or until cooked through and bubbly.

PER SERVING Calories: 336.19 | Fat: 14.09 g | Protein: 18.55 g | Sodium: 140.24 mg | Fiber: 6.11 g | Carbohydrates: 37.13 g | Sugar: 6.20 g

Amazing Minestrone

INGREDIENTS | SERVES 8

4 tablespoons olive oil

5 garlic cloves

2 yellow onions, chopped

2 cups chopped celery

2 cups chopped carrots

4 cups filtered water

4 cups tomato sauce

2 zucchini, chopped

2 cups green beans, chopped

1 cup soaked kidney beans

1 cup soaked white beans

2 cups baby spinach leaves

1 tablespoon oregano

2 tablespoons chopped basil

1 teaspoon all-natural sea salt

1 teaspoon freshly ground black pepper

1. In a large pot over medium heat, sauté 1 tablespoon of olive oil, garlic, onion, celery, and carrots for 8–10 minutes.

2. Add the water and the tomato sauce to the pot, and bring to a boil.

3. Reduce heat to low and add the zucchini, green beans, kidney beans, white beans, spinach leaves, and spices. Simmer on low for 1–2 hours.

4. Serve the soup by itself or over cooked whole-wheat shell pasta.

PER SERVING Calories: 282.81 | Fat: 7.59 g | Protein: 13.50 g | Sodium: 1002.04 mg | Fiber: 14.70 g | Carbohydrates: 43.85 g | Sugar: 11.60 g

Creamy Asparagus Soup

INGREDIENTS | SERVES 4

1 tablespoon olive oil

1 garlic clove

2 small Idaho potatoes, peeled and chopped

2 tablespoons filtered water

2 pounds asparagus, chopped

3 leeks, cleaned and chopped

2 teaspoons freshly ground black pepper

2 cups almond milk

1. In a stockpot over medium heat, sauté the olive oil, garlic, and potatoes for about 10–15 minutes, adding water as needed to prevent sticking and promote steaming.

2. Add asparagus, leeks, and pepper to the potatoes, and sauté until tender.

3. Add the almond milk to the pot and bring to a boil. Reduce heat to low and simmer for 10–15 minutes.

4. With an immersion blender, emulsify the ingredients until thick and creamy.

PER SERVING Calories: 212.67 | Fat: 3.99 g | Protein: 8.38 g | Sodium: 115.11 mg | Fiber: 9.26 g | Carbohydrates: 35.81 g | Sugar: 8.05 g

Creamy Mushroom and Rice Soup

INGREDIENTS | SERVES 4

4 cups mushrooms, chopped

3 cups filtered water, divided

2 teaspoons minced garlic

2 teaspoons all-natural sea salt

3 teaspoons freshly ground black pepper

2 cups cooked brown rice

1 cup plain Greek-style yogurt

1. In a large pot, sauté the mushrooms in 2–4 tablespoons of the water, the garlic, salt, and pepper for about 5–8 minutes, or until tender.

2. Reduce heat to low, add remaining water, and simmer for about 8–10 minutes.

3. Remove from the heat, add the rice to the pot, and allow to cool.

4. Stir to combine, add the yogurt, and blend well.

PER SERVING Calories: 94.87 | Fat: 0.30 g | Protein: 15.55 g | Sodium: 1247.18 mg | Fiber: 1.15 g | Carbohydrates: 8.87 g | Sugar: 6.33 g

Creamy Broccoli Soup

INGREDIENTS | SERVES 4

3 cups unsweetened almond milk
2 teaspoons all-natural sea salt
2 teaspoons garlic powder
1 teaspoon freshly ground black pepper
2 pounds broccoli florets
1 cup plain low-fat Greek-style yogurt

1. In a large pot over medium heat, bring the almond milk, salt, garlic powder, pepper, and broccoli to a boil. Reduce heat to low and simmer about 10–12 minutes.

2. Remove from heat, and chill for 5 minutes. Using an immersion blender, emulsify the broccoli mixture until no bits remain.

3. Add yogurt ¼ cup at a time, and continue blending with the immersion blender until well blended. Serve hot or cold.

PER SERVING Calories: 148.80 | Fat: 0.86 g | Protein: 13.92 g | Sodium: 1418.14 mg | Fiber: 6.84 g | Carbohydrates: 18.78 g | Sugar: 6.31 g

Fruit Salad with Ginger and Lemon Juice

INGREDIENTS | SERVES 4

1 grapefruit, inside pieces removed
1 cup pineapple chunks
1 cup green seedless grapes, sliced
1 Granny Smith apple, cored, sliced, and chopped
1 cup cubed cantaloupe
1 cup cubed honeydew melon
3 tablespoons freshly squeezed lemon juice
2 tablespoons freshly grated ginger

1. In a mixing bowl, combine the fruit, lemon juice, and grated ginger.

2. Toss to coat and combine thoroughly and share between four salad bowls.

PER SERVING Calories: 126.80 | Fat: 0.55 g | Protein: 1.86 g | Sodium: 18.32 mg | Fiber: 3.22 g | Carbohydrates: 32.25 g | Sugar: 25.32 g

Macaroni Salad with Sautéed Veggies and Vinaigrette

INGREDIENTS | SERVES 4

1 cup yellow pepper slices

1 cup red pepper slices

1 cup yellow onion slices

1 tablespoon olive oil

1 teaspoon all-natural sea salt

2 cups cooked 100% whole-wheat rigatoni

2 tablespoons balsamic vinegar

1. In a large skillet over medium heat, sauté the sliced vegetables with the olive oil and sea salt until tender, about 5 minutes.

2. Remove the peppers and onions from the heat and allow to cool.

3. In a large mixing bowl, combine the rigatoni, tossed veggies, and balsamic until thoroughly combined.

PER SERVING Calories: 206.93 | Fat: 4.34 g | Protein: 6.72 g | Sodium: 598.38 mg | Fiber: 6.75 g | Carbohydrates: 38.15 g | Sugar: 5.47 g

Index

We Have EVERYTHING® on Anything!

The Everything® list spans a wide range of subjects, with more than 500 titles covering 25 different categories:

Business	History	Reference
Careers	Home Improvement	Religion
Children's Storybooks	Everything Kids	Self-Help
Computers	Languages	Sports & Fitness
Cooking	Music	Travel
Crafts and Hobbies	New Age	Wedding
Education/Schools	Parenting	Writing
Games and Puzzles	Personal Finance	
Health	Pets	